Spiritual Childbirth

By Katrina Rasbold

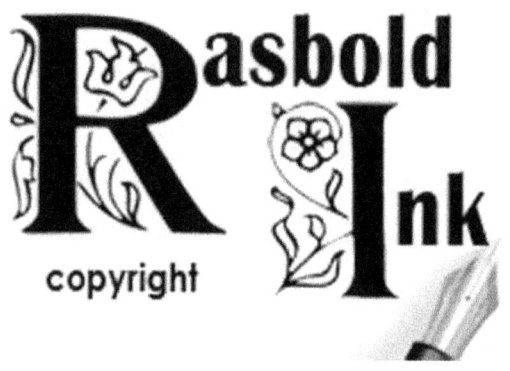

ISBN-13: 978-1499101461

ISBN-10: 1499101465

This book is published by Rasbold Ink: www.rasboldink.com

This book is dedicated to
Christine Thrasher, who
inspired me to write it
and who has been so
enormously patient
as I craft these words.
Christine deserves a beautiful,
spiritual, empowering birth
more than anyone I know.

A very special thanks to
Dr. Karen Albeck who is
my wonderful editor
and works hard to keep
me honest.

TABLE OF CONTENTS

INTRODUCTION

When I had my first child in early 1978 at the age of sixteen, there was no indication of what an important part of my life birth would become over the next few decades. Since time immeasurable, women have bonded over their shared birth stories, but I will not belabor (ha ha) that particular story far beyond simply saying, *"It did not go well."* Twenty-six hours with no training and tremendous pain. The only thing particularly healthy about it was that there was a baby at the end of it.

All of the critical plot points were there, including the biggest blizzard in Kentucky's recorded history closing the road to the hospital. My mother dug her way to the driveway so we could leave and had mild frostbite on her hands when we arrived at the alternative hospital. To hear her tell it, her hands were about to be amputated. I had green paint under my fingernails from clawing the walls in the labor room. I had never seen the doctor who delivered my baby and she was new to the area, so not yet tuned into the hospital. You might as well say, *"Insert epic birth story here."*

I came away from that experience with little interest in ever doing it again, but as many multips know, those sorts of affirmations can mellow over time and in just over two-and-a-half years, I was ready to deliver again, this time at the Navy Regional Medical Center on Guam. One major difference in addition to having the company of a husband for this birth is that we took Lamaze Prepared Childbirth classes.

Even though Lamaze and Bradley practice had already been around since the 1950s and 1960s respectively, in the early 1980s, prepared childbirth was still emerging. My coach and

I practiced dutifully and this time, my labor and delivery was only two hours long. I came out of the experience feeling empowered and excited and I literally telephoned my childbirth instructor, Anna Odahara, from the hospital and said, "Anna, I have to tell people about this. How can I become a childbirth instructor?"

I immediately entered a training program approved by the International Childbirth Education Association and was blessed with wonderful teachers who helped me learn that I was, at my inner core self, a teacher. I know that not many people can say that at the age of eighteen, they began doing what they love doing most in life and continued to do throughout their adult life, but I have been very lucky in that respect. I am still an instructor of a different sort and although I retired from childbirth teaching in 1997, I still act as a Prepared Childbirth Consultant.

In 1982, my approach to childbirth was forever changed. My husband at that time also trained to teach childbirth classes and we began to work as team teachers for a group of midwives called "The Hearth," in Alamogordo, New Mexico. That was our introduction to the wonderful world of home births and we were thrilled to have our third son, Joshua, at home that May. We taught prepared childbirth classes together for several years, which was very rewarding. It was through my work with The Hearth that I first learned that as women, we really can trust our bodies to birth safely and effectively.

I taught classes in England, in California, and in Idaho after that. In California, I began to teach prenatal and breastfeeding classes as well. Throughout this time, I also had the privilege of acting as team support for several laboring couples and women on their own as well.

All through this teaching experience, the power and majesty of birth never failed to bring a tremendous sense of awe to me. In 1992, I gave birth to my daughter at a birthing center in Apple Valley, California where I worked. In 1997 and 1999, I gave birth to two more sons in my home with a group of midwives called "Birthstream" out of Davis, California.

The energy and the "feel" of birth will always be with me. Because we used it as lubrication for perineal massage, extra virgin olive oil still smells like birth to me and probably always will. I sleep with a pillow between my knees as I taught my pregnant students. I Kegel every day and keep a tennis ball at my desk for muscle massage.

During our home birth training back in the early 1980s, I read a book called *Spiritual Midwifery* by a wonderful woman named Ina May Gaskin (right), who was extremely formative in revising my mindset regarding birth with her frank and unaffected writing. She introduced the spiritual component of birth that my training had not covered to that point and that my personal experience had barely touched. So intent had I been on the

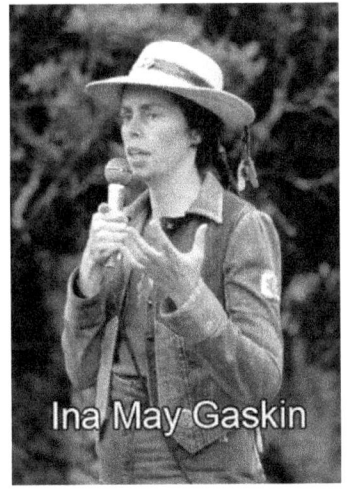

Ina May Gaskin

physiological and pain-reducing aspects of birth that I had never considered what a monumentally spiritual experience pregnancy and childbirth can be when approached with that focus in mind.

Of course, birth has been a spiritual experience since women first began to birth. We were worshipped, adored, admired, and feared for our ability to produce life. Society often takes for granted the amazing fact that a woman can grow a whole new person inside her and once she starts pushing, in very little time there are two people where before there was only one.

Not only can a woman create another person, but she can then manifest the most perfect food to feed that new life. The process is occasionally broken, sure, but as a whole, it is quite efficient and impressive.

In the intervening years between 1982 and my sixth child's birth in 1999, I immersed myself into the idea of birth as a spiritual expression of feminine power. My first two years of training on Guam took place in hospitals with nurses as my teachers. They gave me a good starting point, but their perception of birth was warped by their career and cohort choice.

For instance, I used to actually teach that *"Forceps do not pull on the baby's head but instead, simply push the imposing vaginal canal away from the baby so that it can emerge naturally."* Imagine my great surprise when I witnessed my first forceps birth! Much of the class I taught in my first two years of instruction was hospital propaganda such as that, which I taught simply because it was what I was told to say and therefore, believed to be true.

We were on the edge of change when hospitals were only beginning to "allow" laboring women to have support people with them. The year I began teaching, police arrested a man in New York for handcuffing himself to his wife who was in advanced labor. His charge? *Trespassing.* Women were restrained in birth to keep them from reaching up onto their own bellies to touch their babies and thereby contaminating the sterile field. Their legs were stirrupped into the air at right angles to their bodies for the ease of the delivering doctor's access, not for any thought of the woman's comfort in delivering.

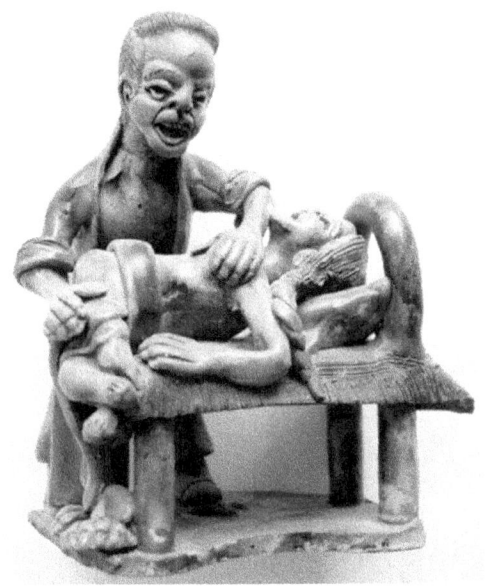

Peruvian statue of a man attending a woman in childbirth

Vaginas were cut for every birth because forceps were used for nearly every birth and the position of the stirrups drew the perineum tight over the baby's head allowing the vaginal and perineal tissues no flexibility of movement. The message this sent to women was, "Your body must be surgically enhanced because it is incapable of giving birth naturally. Be grateful we are here to do this for you or you and your baby would die."

When a laboring woman was admitted to the hospital, she was immediately tethered to an IV drip so that medication could be administered very quickly and so she could be hydrated as she was allowed no drink and no sustenance for her time in the hospital other than spoonfuls of ice chips. Can you imagine going into the most intense athletic event of your life with no nourishment other than slivers of ice?

The administration of medication was presumed rather than used "as needed." I actually watched a nurse chase the gurney down the hall of the hospital as staff wheeled a woman into the delivery room. Why was she chasing the gurney? So she could push a large dose of Demerol into the laboring woman's IV. The woman's labor progressed rapidly and by the time she was on the gurney and moving, the *baby's head was already crowning* but *oh no! She hadn't gotten her Demerol yet!!*

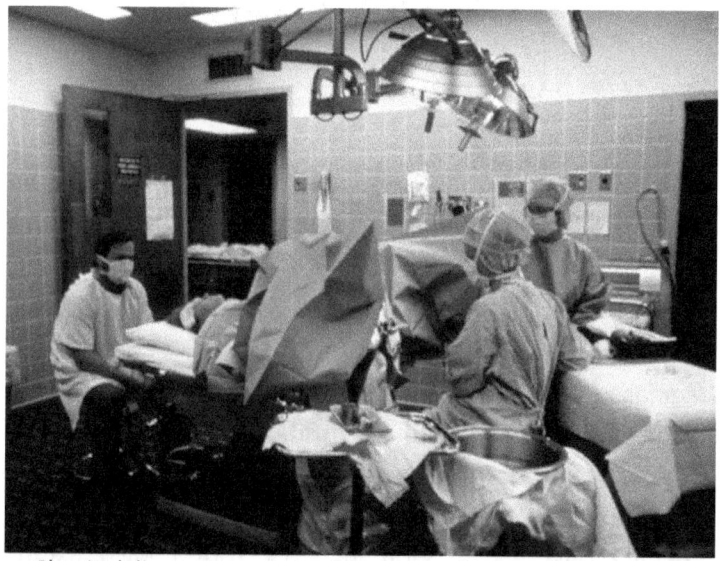

*Classic delivery room set up for a **normal** birth. Those are the mother's legs up in the air under those drapes. The anesthetist is ready at her head to administer anesthesia. Mom looks empowered, right?*

So indoctrinated was the hospital staff that they still rushed to insert an IV line and push analgesics, even though that baby was out and breastfeeding within fifteen minutes, *which was when the Demerol began to take effect.* We have enjoyed *tremendous* progress in the reform of the birth process in hospitals, yet no matter how effectively and magnificently a woman's body works to birth her baby, most hospitals still cling to the premise that birth is an emergency medical crisis waiting to happen rather than a natural process.Upon admission in those days, a laboring woman was given what was called a "Triple H" enema, which meant "High, Hot, and Hell of a lot." The flow of water into the rectum aggressively stimulated the contracting uterus through the thin rectal wall, causing erratic and intense contractions. The uterus is a muscular organ that is extremely sensitive to stimulation. If you press on a pregnant woman's belly in the area of her uterus, assuming she is thirty weeks or more pregnant, you can see and feel her uterus tense and pull up within a minute or two. This is in response to the stimulation of touch and in that case is through much more body tissue than the thin rectal wall. The rush of water from the enema sent the contracting uterus into a state of hyperstimulation. Additionally, the bearing down sensation the enema created could bruise the malleable cervix since most women are unable to differentiate between rectal and pelvic pushing. Another concern is that enemas cause liquid fecal matter to contact the lower part of the body, including the vagina.

The public hair of women was shaved for sterility even though no practice related to birth involves the pubic mons. The inevitable nicks and cuts that occurred while trying to shave the pubic hair of laboring women often became painfully infected and the itchy regrowth added discomfort to the postnatal recovery period.

From the time she was admitted to the hospital, the laboring woman was restricted to the bed and had to stay on her back to allow for external fetal monitoring. When pregnant women lie on their backs for more than a few minutes, compression of the superior vena cava, which carries blood flow to the brain and to the baby, occurs from the weight of the baby and the uterus. This reduction in blood flow causes the mother to become weak, nauseated, and dizzy and the baby's heart tones to slow down. Hospital staff considered these side effects to be complications of labor rather than a simple postural issue and most often, they were managed surgically or with medication as a state of emergency rather than simply rolling the mother onto her left side, which corrects both problems immediately.

When I began teaching, women sometimes received a drug called "Scopolamine," which was a favorite at the time because after the birth, they remembered nothing that occurred while they labored and delivered. The drug was an amnesiac that produced what doctors called "twilight sleep" in which the mother was, in theory, half-awake and half-asleep. The amnesiac qualities caused the mothers to have no memory of what happened during their birth; however, the drug was also a strong hallucinogenic and they would often experience horrific delusions of spiders, snakes, and other nightmarish things. Women on Scopolamine often thought the staff was trying to kill them as it can cause extreme paranoia and disorientation. Use of this medication required that a woman be restrained to the bed during labor for her own protection, as well as the staff's. Imagine walking into a labor room and seeing a screaming, terrified, laboring woman with her arms and feet tied to the four corners of the bed and now imagine that this happened well within the past few decades.

Even in our "enlightened" transitional time during the early 1980s, we considered ourselves lucky that women could begin pushing their babies out in the labor room rather than the entire birth taking place in the uncomfortable delivery room. They still had to be transitioned to the delivery room for actual birth, but until crowning, when the largest part of the baby's head passes under the mother's pubic archway, she pushed in the labor room. This means that at the height of the birthing process when her urge to push is most overwhelming, the mother had to *stop pushing* for some time, usually fifteen to twenty minutes, while she was moved onto a gurney, then into the delivery room, then moved onto the delivery table to be strapped down for the birth.

It was a big deal for us when the labor beds could be rolled directly into the delivery room, omitting the transition onto the gurney. Then the mother only had one butt leap from the labor bed to the delivery table. We used to have women practice moving their butt first onto the delivery table by having them take off their shoe and lay it next to their butt long ways, then heaving their pregnant selves over the shoe.

If you have had any experience with birth in the past five to ten years, you know that these practices seem out of the dark ages compared to current birthing routines. In most quality hospitals at the time of this writing, greater consideration is giving to the laboring mother's comfort, her support team, and her pre-birth planning interests.

I mention these ridiculous routines because they happened during our generation and are not that far removed from us. For hundreds of years, women have had their births medically managed rather than joyfully experienced, which has colored how society views human birth. Those who chose other paths, such as home birth, were, and are sometimes still, seen as the lunatic fringe. Anyone who was assertive about their birth choices in outlining specific requests to their obstetrician were considered the "problem children." Only those who smiled and said yes to all routine hospital policies were on the "good girl list."

How in the world could something as clinical and invasive, working against the very nature and physiological process of birth, inspire any sort of spiritual aspect? It was only when women began to reclaim the process of birth as their own that they were able to find their inner Goddess. Only then could they embrace the strength and empowerment that is their birthright in the birthing process.

Often, so much emphasis falls on the physical comfort of the mother and medical management of the birth that little, if any, attention reaches the spiritual aspect of the birth process in the hospital environment. I have seen it as a more prominent factor in home birth and midwife facilitated births, but it is up to the laboring mother and her caretakers to awaken and strengthen this connection.

The fact is that a hospital is *not* set up as a place to treat conditions of health, but to manage and cure conditions of illness. Birth is the *ultimate* expression of health and yet many medical professionals still treat it as a disease. Despite the fact that only approximately 10-15% of births have complications that involve medical intervention, both expectant parents and maternity staff still approach it as an emergency waiting to happen. Our cesarean rate is currently at approximately 32%, which is far beyond that 10-15% range of complication.

Some of this is, like the complications I mentioned previously that come from a laboring woman being confined to a bed on her back, the result of previous interventions. Most often, I have found that it is because of what *might* go wrong next. Interestingly, as high as our national cesarean section rate might be, it is not the worst. In China, the rate is 46%. China embraces a practice that is becoming more popular in the United States, which is an elective cesarean with no medical necessity.

In many cases, as described above, medical intervention in childbirth is a chain reaction of complications. A doctor is uncomfortable with a woman going a week beyond her due date and she is weary and ready to be finished being pregnant. They schedule an induction. The medical staff breaks her water and labor does not begin. She now must complete the childbirth within forty-eight hours because of the risk of infection, so they give her Pitocin to stimulate contractions artificially, which is a very painful process. Her cervix is not yet ripe enough to dilate effectively because she was not actually supposed to go into labor naturally for another week, so she does not progress in cervical dilation. She becomes exhausted and the baby begins to go into distress, so they perform a cesarean section and the result is that everyone is grateful that medical intervention was there to keep the mother and baby safe. Had they monitored the baby's heart tones and movement and the mother's blood pressure and waited until she went into labor naturally, she possibly could have had a healthy vaginal birth.

One of the greatest insults to womankind is the odd, conditioned belief that our bodies are not to be trusted to birth our babies and that childbirth is a state of impending emergency. For centuries, we put our own power of birth into the hands of men. We relinquished our greatest gift, our strongest empowerment, because we bought into the lie that our births need to be managed by the males of the tribe rather than our sisters, our mothers, and our midwives.

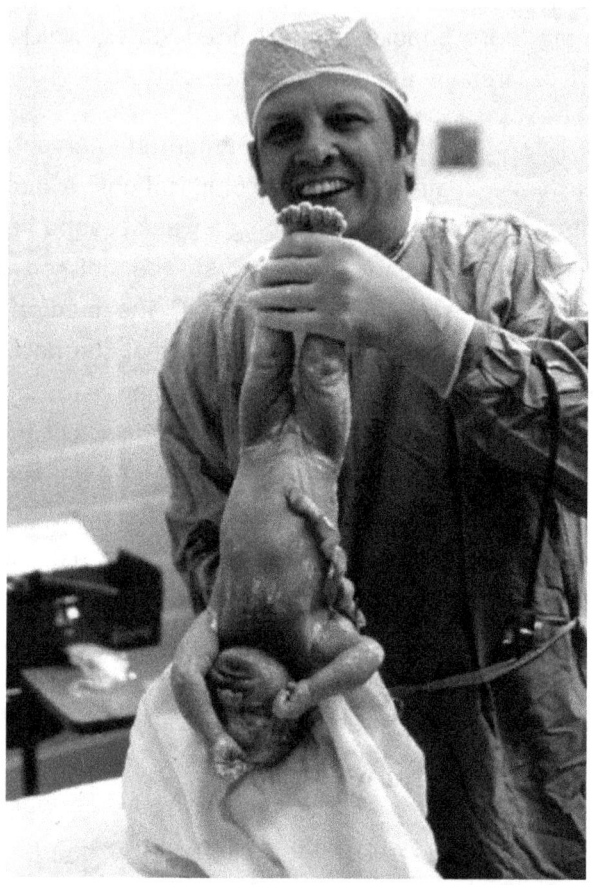

A physician holds up a baby immediately after delivery by cesarean section in Minnesota in 1974.

Notice even how the terminology changed. We say that a woman "was delivered of" a healthy baby boy or that "Dr. So and So delivered my baby." The mother is seen as little more than a fleshy tunnel the baby passes through as the doctor brings it into life. The fact that she has grown this baby within her and that *she* is now the one delivering it into the world has been completely lost, even in our progressive era. The correct answer to the question, "Who delivered your baby?" is "I did."

In the previous photo, you will notice the baby is unconscious due to heavy sedation of the mother with general anesthesia. You will also notice the doctor holds up the baby like a trophy fish in a sportsman's magazine. The effect of heavy medication on the newborn is what started the practice of "spanking" a newborn so the pain created by striking the baby would bring it back to consciousness.

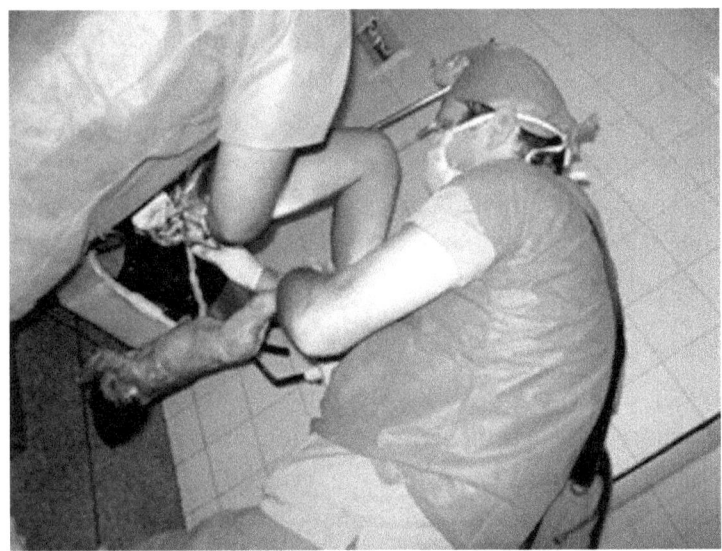

The practice of holding babies up by the heels is now strongly discouraged because the baby has spent its entire life in a curled position inside the womb as it floats weightlessly in fluid. Forcing the hips to support the weight of the baby immediately after birth sometimes caused hip displacement, which the hospitals believed was a congenital deformity, rather than caused by their own routine practices. In the above photo, the baby is extremely bloody from the cut required in the lower vagina when a woman delivers her baby while in stirrups.

Am I a She-Ra, man hating, Femi-Nazi? Absolutely not! I love men. Men are some of my favorite living things on earth. I love male energy and I love seeing a man in his full empowerment...just as I love seeing a woman in her full empowerment. Those energies complement one another perfectly. There is no denying, however, that centuries of patriarchal oppression in which society treated women as no more than chattel like goats or shovels, still defines many of our common behaviors in society, including our birth practices over the past century.

Do I despise and shun Westernized medicine? That is a more complicated question. I am grateful for medical expertise when it is needed, but I do feel that there should be far greater patient responsibility in terms of education and tuning into one's body rather than blindly turning over the entirety of your physical care to another person or institution.

When my mother had a brain tumor the size of a lemon, I was grateful beyond measure for the medical care that diagnosed and removed the tumor. When I decided I needed to put a stop to my baby having, I was thrilled that I could safely have a tubal ligation. I was thankful for the reassurance doctors and nurse practitioners sometimes gave me that I was doing the right things when my children were ill.

There is a balance between the gifts and blessings of professional medical expertise and personal health care responsibilities. Too often simple illness or injury results in hysteria and panic rather than calmly treating the problem. Our bodies are well equipped to tell us exactly what it needs if we educate ourselves about nutrition and learn our body's own rhythms. We can learn how much sleep we personally need for optimum health and focus rather than statistical standards, what types of foods work best with our own digestive system to keep us strong and healthy, and what kind of exercise our body responds to best. We can learn our sensitivities to different foods like dairy, gluten, proteins, carbohydrates, and fats. The more we get to know our own physical needs, and our own bodies, the closer we come to taking responsibility for our health and wellness.

This extends to pregnancy as well. There was a time when women came to a midwife when they had a problem with their pregnancy that they needed to discuss or they were in labor. Prenatal monitoring to the level that we now experience is a relatively new process. All through their pregnancies, women are screened for rare conditions on the off chance that they might be there. This, again, creates a feeling of brokenness and helplessness in the pregnant woman; as though she cannot be trusted to incubate her baby successfully without falling victim to a huge laundry list of possible afflictions.

I hasten to point out that those women of the past who did not have regular prenatal care also lived their lives in the company of many other women, most of whom experienced birth to a degree that we do not in our modern society. They gave birth more often and started doing so earlier. They were used to supporting one another throughout pregnancy and childbirth and formed a tremendous support system. When a woman went into labor, her friends, sisters, aunts, mother, and other women who were familiar with the birthing process surrounded her and supported her through the experience. Without that positive support throughout pregnancy and birth and certainly without that many eyes on the pregnant mother, monitoring her eating, her drinking, her exercise, and her behavior, routine professional prenatal care became essential.

Throughout time, women spoke of their births as triumphant undertakings. Now, the stories are often about an ominous sense of impending danger and mostly focus on what went *wrong* rather than what went *right*. Women wear their complications of childbirth like Girl Scout merit badges.

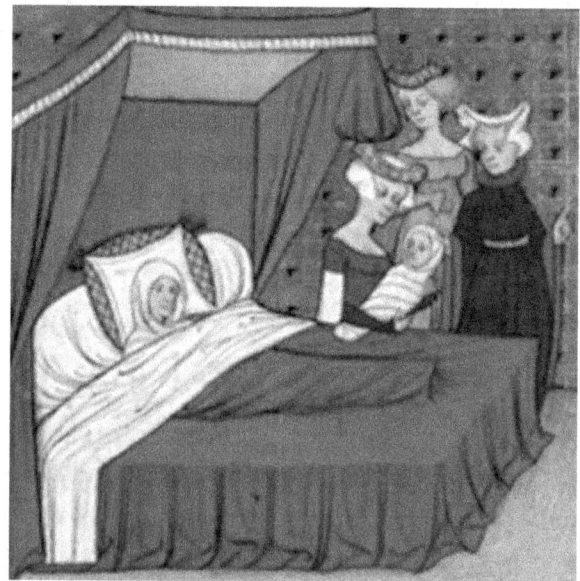

Not one dude in sight

When birth was treated by women as a natural process, our minds, bodies, and spirits worked together to create that outcome. When the focus is on fear, danger, and impending doom, our attention will often create *that* outcome.

What we focus on grows.

In today's maternity world, we have a good grasp of the "body" aspect of the mind-body-spirit trinity with advanced understanding of how the birthing process functions and how to make laboring mothers as comfortable as possible. The "mind" aspect gets attention from the current practice of allowing friends, family, and her partner to act as a support team during labor and delivery, as well as providing quality education about the birth process and pain managing techniques.

The only area still left unmanaged is that of spirit, which is why I wrote this book. Women have so distanced themselves away from the birthing process that a healthy, uncomplicated birth feels neither natural nor achievable to many pregnant women. A return to the natural process of birth where a woman not only has confidence in her ability to birth, but also views it as a spiritual gift is the final integration of mind, body, and spirit into the childbirth process.

My mother used to say that with her first baby, a woman is afraid because she does not know what to expect and with her next baby, she is afraid because she does know what to expect. It is comments like these on which our daughters form their opinion of birthing, one of the most phenomenal experiences they will ever have.

Rarely does a woman receive from health care professionals or her cohorts the confidence that she can deliver a healthy, strong baby with ease. The midwives with whom I worked were the most open to instilling that idea into their clients and I have found this often to be the case with midwives. For the pregnant woman who wishes fully exploring the spirituality of birth, I whole-heartedly recommend researching midwives in your area and if possible, securing personal recommendations.

The word "midwife" translates out to "with woman" and is about simply staying with a woman during her birth.

Midwives of today are trained to handle all manner of birthing complications when they do arise, but most will tell you that their rate of complications is significantly lower than their hospital-based counterparts.

The most logical reason for these very different statistics is that most high-risk pregnancies do not have the option of using a midwife for delivery and must transfer to a higher level of medical management. It has been my experience, however, that a great deal of the tremendous success midwives have in turning out remarkable statistics of healthy births with minimal intervention comes directly from their near universal ability to wait patiently while a woman's body figures out what it is doing and to provide positive, life-affirming support during the pregnancy and childbirth process.

Many midwives care for the laboring and delivering woman in her own home, so she is more relaxed and calm. The process of relocating to a medical facility for birth can be traumatic, especially if labor is progressing quickly. At home, she does not have to adjust to new surroundings or sequester away from the people she loves.

Most midwives allow their clients a broad spectrum of control over their own birthing process, conducting extensive interviews to learn what the woman wants for her birth plan and how best to meet her needs. They emphasize education and help women to learn the physiological processes of childbirth and effective pain management techniques.

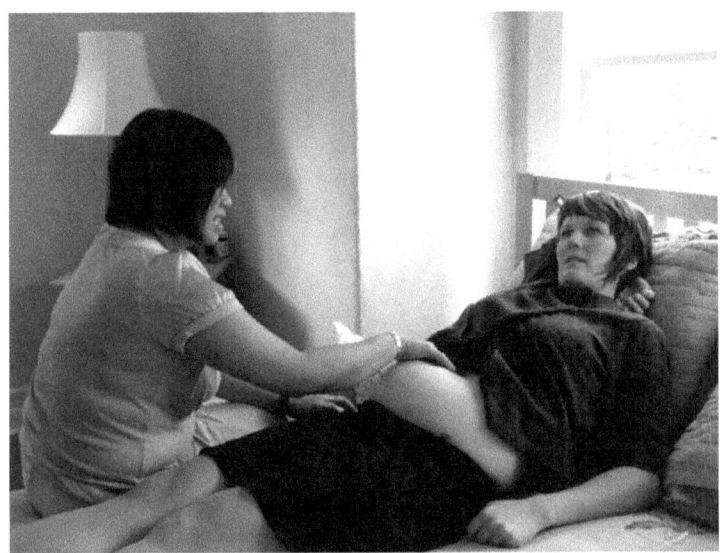
When a woman is afforded the respect of having all of her questions about her body and her birth answered and when she feels safe and informed, it is far easier for her to access the spiritual side of birth and to going to the process with confidence, whether this is achieved through home birth, hospital birth, or birthing center birth.

Home birth with midwives is an amazing experience, but it is not one suited to every woman and every pregnancy. As mentioned before, some women have high-risk pregnancies that require closer observation and greater access to emergency equipment. Today's midwives are increasingly capable of handling birthing emergencies, but some unique complications such as a placenta that is not well-placed, extremely high blood pressure, or multiple births can pose greater risk and are not considered by most professionals to be good candidates for a home birth.

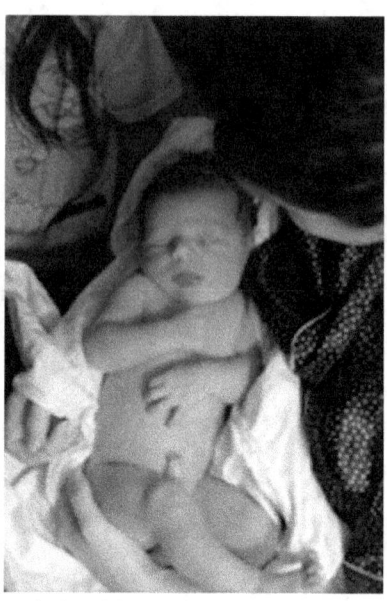

*A baby delivered at home, looking
remarkably like a baby delivered
in the hospital. (That kid is HUGE!)*

Some women are frightened of birth to the point that they cannot labor comfortably unless they are in a hospital. Each person must take the circumstances of their own pregnancy and emotional well-being into deep consideration when planning their place of birth. Likewise, they must carefully consider who will be on their birthing support team and make their choices based not on the expectations of others or a sense of obligation, but on what is best for the laboring mother. A good example of this is when a grandmother insists on being in the room for the birth of her grandchild, but has a contentious relationship with the laboring mother, her partner, or both. Tensions such as these have no place in the birthing environment. The mother's emotional well-being and sense of security are of the utmost concern when making choices such as these. She should never feel that she has to play hostess or referee while laboring.

Whether you choose to birth at home, in a birthing center, or in a hospital, you must make the decision that works best for you and not necessarily for others. The goal is to search your heart, find what birthing plan best suits your own unique needs, and then create a dedicated support team of loved ones and professionals who develop and work toward that outcome.

In today's world, many expectant mothers are excited about approaching pregnancy and childbirth as a spiritual journey rather than simply a medical one. Knowing that they will likely only give birth a scant few times in their lives, they wish to make it a significant and personal process that tunes them into the cycles and processes of nature in a particularly profound way.

While there are many books that detail the medical side of birth, this one included, a major difference is that *Spiritual Childbirth* will also explore the energy of birth and its sacred aspects.

Within this text, you will find adult discussions about body parts, body functions, and life experiences. We will follow the birthing process from fertilization, through pregnancy, and into labor and delivery. We will discuss routine medical procedures you can expect with normal childbirth, complications of childbirth and their levels of medical management, and emergency childbirth for unexpected delivery away from your chosen place of birth.

Will we not only cover those individual subjects in detail, but also explore the spiritual significance of the process and learn how to instill a sacred awareness into each step of the birthing experience. By taking an active role in embracing the spiritual side of birth, you join a revolution that has been underway for decades devoted to returning the power of the birthing process to the women who so richly deserve it.

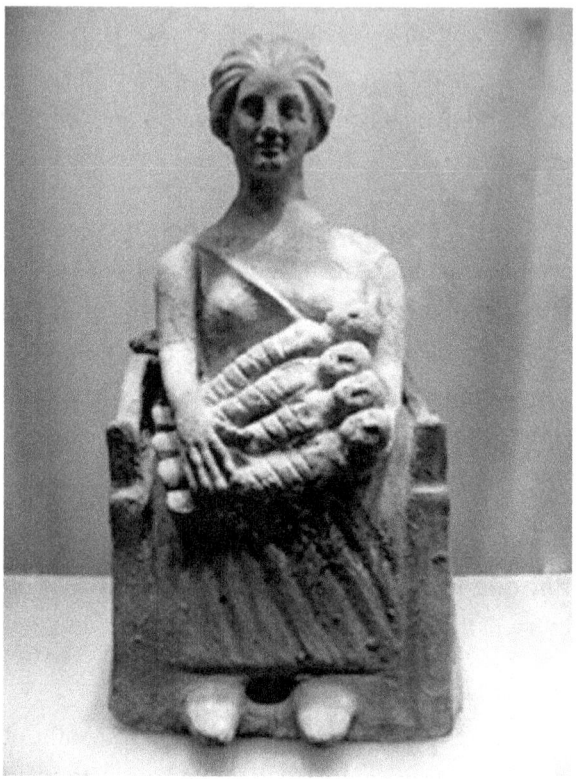

CHAPTER 1 – CONCEPTION AND CONTRACEPTION

Fertilization & Conception

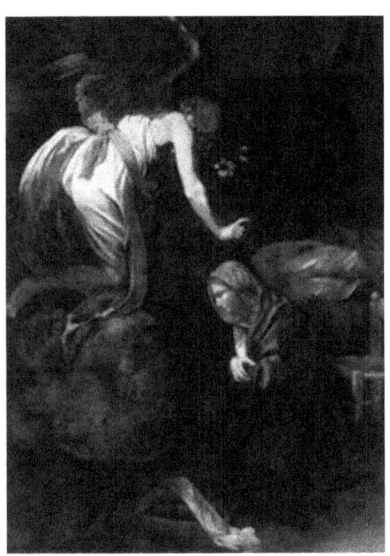

As many of us know well, a frequent side effect of sex is pregnancy. Most of us have a time when we feel bulletproof and believe that we will not become pregnant "this one time." Many of us go through attempts to become pregnant and feel that wave of disappointment when that period comes yet again. I have personally gotten pregnant on very nearly every birth control method on the market and some that are even no longer on the market.

I found out I was pregnant with my third son the week my husband at that time had his vasectomy. I found out I was pregnant with my fifth son through the pre-operative testing to rule out pregnancy *three days before my tubal ligation*. I got pregnant with my daughter using a condom and a sponge on the last day of my period. One of my babies was a "bulletproof theory" baby. Two were planned. Three were "despite all odds and being very responsible."

The insensitivity of people around women who have more than the usual two point five children is unbelievable. I heard everything from "Guess you haven't figured out what is causing it, have you?" to "You are just breeder stock, huh?" to "They have this thing called birth control..." The fact that I chose to welcome an unexpected baby rather than reject it for some reason elicited harsh and hurtful criticism from others. People feel compelled, for reasons I cannot imagine, to insinuate themselves into the fertility choices of others.

Regardless, it all starts with: Sex. *Or does it?*

One would think that a person always has to have sex in order to conceive, but there have been instances in which women have actually conceived without penetration. In vitro fertilization or even artificial insemination is likely the first thing a person considers, but while infertility and the means of becoming pregnant through alternative procedures is a worthy subject, in this case, I am talking about women who conceived without medical intervention and also without having actual intercourse.

Although myths abound about women conceiving from toilet seats or a bath sponge they shared with a partner, it is important to know that although sperm can live for five to seven days inside a body under ideal conditions, on the outside, the shelf life of sperm is only around twenty minutes at best. As soon as sperm encounter the outside world, they begin to deteriorate and their mobility is greatly compromised. This means that even in the twenty minutes or so before they die, they are not in ideal or even viable impregnating condition. They do not lie in wait for an unsuspecting vagina and then storm the gates with a battering ram. This is why sperm samples are usually collected onsite rather than at home. There is also a frequent saliva contamination on sperm samples drawn at home. (Ahem)

With the twenty minute death knell tolling, sperm that are not introduced directly into the vagina have to work extra hard to reach the fertilization point. It can, however, be done if conditions are very specific.

The most common form of "virgin birth" is when a couple engages in active foreplay and although penetration does not occur, ejaculation takes place near the vaginal opening (with or without panties present). In this case, semen can leak into the vaginal opening, carrying sperm along with it.

When I was training as a childbirth instructor, a lecturing physician told us about a case he encountered in which a woman presented to the emergency room in obvious profound physical distress. She was clearly in the advanced stages of pregnancy and in active labor. When the staff attempted to examine her vaginally to determine her progression, they found to their surprise that she had no vaginal opening. (?!)

They performed an emergency cesarean and both mother and baby were healthy. Upon interviewing the patient, the staff learned that the women had been born without a vaginal opening and never had corrective surgery and therefore *had never had intercourse* and yet, pregnant she was. Of course, there was a story behind this one.

At the time of the conception of her child, the woman was caught performing oral sex on another woman's husband. The wife walked in on the scene at the exact moment of ejaculation and, as so often happens at special moments such as these, a knife fight ensued. The patient received a stab wound that lacerated her abdomen and stomach. She was rushed to the hospital and the wound was surgically repaired. The wound went through her abdomen and perforated her stomach, spilling the contents of her stomach into her abdominal cavity.

When she was in surgery, the abdominal cavity was irrigated and cleaned; however, by that time, the semen from her stomach had leaked into her abdominal cavity and sperm made their way into the uterus from the inside. The patient stayed in denial about her pregnancy until the onset of labor because in her mind, she had never had penetrative sex and therefore, could not possibly be pregnant.

The act of conception seems so easy for some and so difficult for others. In reality, it is like salmon swimming upstream. It is a battle against the odds that is won or lost. Here are the basic mechanics of fertilization and this time, we will presume that actual sex was involved.

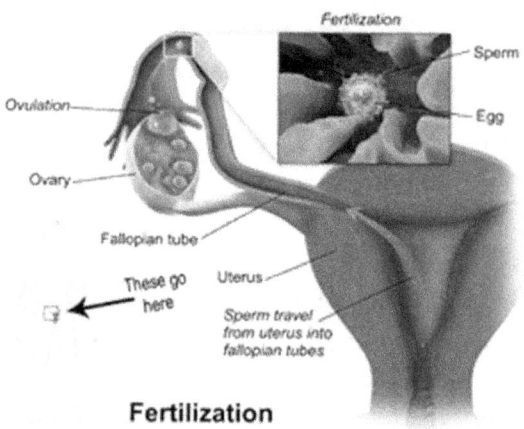

Fertilization

These are the female reproductive organs. The uterus is about the size of your fist and shaped like an inverted pear. The top of the uterus is called the fundus and the bottom, which is a bottleneck like projection, is called the cervix. The external os (opening) is at the very middle of the outer end of the cervix and the internal os is at the top end of the cervix, opening into the uterine cavity. Another more archaic word for uterus is "womb."

Each month, most fertile women will produce an egg from one of their ovaries. Typically, the ovaries alternate in releasing the egg. A blister, called a follicle, will form on the ovary and an egg will burst forth from that follicle. At this point, the egg is unfertilized and the woman is not yet pregnant; she has merely ovulated. This usually happens on the fourteenth day after the first day of her last menstrual period.

Remember that sperm can remain vital in the woman's body for five to seven days after ejaculation. Although the egg remains available for fertilization for only seventy-two hours or so after its release, a woman can still become pregnant if she does not have sex during those three days. If she had sex a few days before she ovulated, there may still be living, active sperm in the vaginal cavity, uterus and/or fallopian tubes lying in wait for the newly released egg.

On each side of the uterus between the fundus and the ovary, there is a fallopian tube. It is wider at the ovarian end than it is at the uterine end. Once the ovary releases the egg, hair-like projections inside the fallopian tubes called cilia begin to draw the egg up into the fallopian tubes. The cilia move rhythmically, which creates a suction-type action that moves the egg up into the tube on the side closest to the releasing ovary. It is common for a woman to feel a slight cramping sensation when the egg releases. The new egg begins to travel inside the fallopian tube from the wider end where it entered toward the narrower end that will eventually drop it out into the uterus, fertilized or unfertilized.

In the tablespoon or so of semen that is released when a man ejaculates, there are between one hundred million and six hundred million or so sperm. Sperm counts vary dramatically from man to man. On the typical vaginal intercourse session, ejaculation will occur on the down stroke, which neatly delivers the bulk of semen right to the outer os of the cervix. The vaginal environment is enormously hostile to the sperm and immediately begins killing them off. There is usually a large number of malformed sperm (two heads, two tails, crooked backs, etc) that begin immediately and foolishly running into walls and never really getting anywhere productive.

When the remaining sperm successfully reach the cervical opening of the ovulating or near-ovulating woman, they have a stronger chance of survival. There is an increase of cervical mucus around the time of ovulation and the mucus is very hospitable to the sperm after their battle through the vaginal battleground. The sperm begin to swim upward into the uterus and find the small end of the fallopian tube that connects to the fundus of the uterus. By this time, the numbers of healthy, vital sperm have diminished significantly so that only a few hundred thousand are actually able to enter the fallopian tube. We must also consider that around half of these remaining viable sperm will go barreling into the wrong fallopian tube where there is no egg waiting. [Insert joke here about asking for directions.]

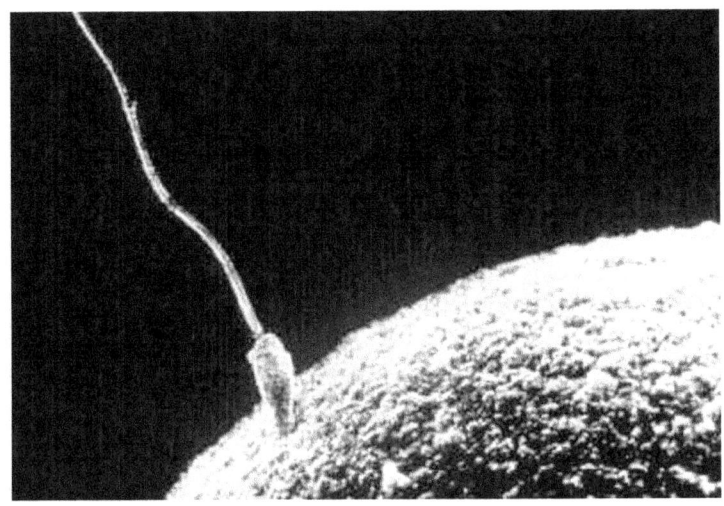

As soon as the sperm intersect the egg, they begin aggressively attempting to penetrate the outer protective covering of the egg. Although many may penetrate the outer layer, only one will make it into the inner sanctum of the egg. Once that penetration occurs, the egg flies into action and the outer layer hardens, preventing more than one sperm from penetrating the inner nucleus of the egg cell.

The hardening of the outer shell causes the tail of the sperm to break off so that the head of the successful sperm and the egg now create a two-celled organism called a zygote. Immediately, those two cells divide into four cells. Each cell begins to double repeatedly at such an astounding rate that the momentum of the movement of cell division creates a rolling effect and the fertilized egg, also propelled by the fallopian tube cilia, begins to move into the smaller end of the fallopian tube and into the uterus.

The fertilized egg, then called a blastocyst, free falls into the uterine cavity and lands on the soft, spongy wall of the uterus. It burrows into the wall of the uterus and is then called an embryo. That soft, spongy uterine lining would have been the woman's menstrual period had she not conceived. If no conception occurs, the uterine lining sheds and a new one grows each month. The entire process from fertilization until implantation takes approximately six to twelve days.

How Birth Control Works

Now that you know how fertilization and conception takes place, it is easier to understand how different method of birth control work (or do not):

Rhythm Methods (also called "Natural Family Planning") involve abstaining from sex or using a barrier form of birth control, during the week or so out of the month when a woman is likely to conceive. The woman's menstruation and ovulation are carefully charted. Her basal body temperature is monitored for slight spikes that occur around ovulation and her cervical mucus is regularly checked for thickening.

Barrier Methods attempt to keep the sperm and egg from meeting. These include condoms, diaphragms, cervical caps, and other methods that block access. For optimal protection, it is important to use a chemical method in addition to the barrier method.

Chemical Methods attempt to eliminate sperm with spermicide, usually in foam or jelly form. These are introduced into the vagina near the cervical os prior to sex. The diaphragm and the sponge use both a barrier method and a spermicide.

Anti-Ovulant Methods fool the body into thinking it is pregnant by releasing hormones into the bloodstream that mimic pregnancy. A woman does not ovulate during pregnancy and so no egg is released. This method includes birth control pills, shots, patches, and implants.

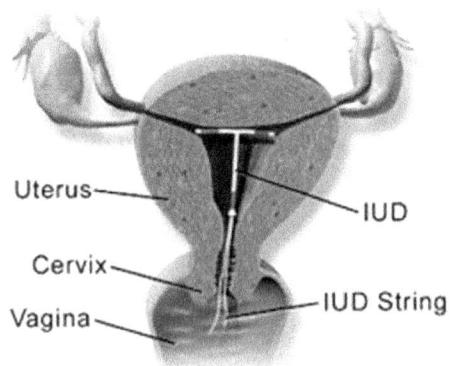

Intrauterine Device

Uterine Implant Methods introduce a foreign body called an IUD (Intrauterine Device) through the cervix and into the uterine cavity during a doctor's exam. The small plastic or copper device remains in the uterus and irritates the wall of the uterus enough that the fertilized egg is unable to implant. The fertilized egg is then absorbed or discharged by the body rather than implanting.

Surgical Methods are available for males or females. In the female (a bilateral tubal ligation or "BTL"), a surgeon makes two incisions into the woman's abdomen: one in the navel and one above the public bone. A laparoscope goes into the navel incision and a manipulating probe into the pubic incision. The woman's fallopian tubes are tied off, cut, and cauterized. This prevents the ovulated egg entering the fallopian tube to encounter the sperm.

In the male (a vasectomy), the vas deferens tubes are cut and cauterized, which keeps the sperm from ever entering semen. Semen still releases and the sensation is identical during orgasm; however, there is no sperm in the semen. The male essentially, "shoots blanks."

Of these contraceptive measures, surgical methods are the most reliable. Although they are surgically reversible, a person should never make the decision to be sterilized unless they are certain they do not wish to have children and should consider either of these a permanent procedure. Since the abdominal wall is breached during the tubal ligation, it is more medically invasive surgery when compared to the vasectomy. Recovery time is typically two weeks and the woman must receive either a general anesthetic or a spinal anesthetic.

The vasectomy is often more emotionally difficult due to the protective feelings many men have toward their male anatomy. The vasectomy is done under a local anesthetic with a mild sedative (a 50-mg. Valium tablet is common) given orally an hour or two before the surgery. Recovery time is usually forty-eight to seventy-two hours. In the case of a vasectomy, it is advisable to use a back-up form of birth for up to two weeks after the procedure (or a certain number of ejaculates) to allow for flushing out of sperm already present in the semen prior to the surgery.

An interesting fact is that many physicians and medical groups still have the policy that they will not perform a tubal ligation on a woman until she is of a specific age, usually twenty-five, or has a certain number of children; however, they will perform a vasectomy on a man at any age or circumstance.

Ineffective methods include douching with any variety of substances. Douching is actually recommended as a fertility method since it hydroplanes the sperm toward the cervix faster. Other ineffective methods are "doing it standing up," standing up immediately afterwards, aspirin in a coke, withdrawal or "pulling out," condoms or spermicidal agents alone, and methods that sit in a drawer unused.

The Spiritual Aspect of Fertilization, Conception, and Contraception

One might not believe that there is a spiritual side to contraception, but when we look at the bigger picture, it is easy to see. Until the advent of patriarchal dominance, women long took control over their reproductive choices by using herbs and energy movement. It was only for a brief time that a woman's reproductive activities were not within her control.

The power to give life is one most women hold dear and I know very few who abuse that power. We all know people who are not particularly maternal, but for the most part, the enormity of what they are doing as they gestate and birth tends to hit home at some point or another.

When Margaret Sanger coined the phrase "birth control" in the early 1900s, she started a revolution of women refusing to accept back alley abortions as their only recourse for managing their own fertility. She worked aggressively with every class of woman under the motto of "No Gods, No Masters," and insisted that every woman was "mistress of her own body." This enraged the reigning paradigm and she ultimately was arrested under the Comstock Law for distributing information on contraception.

She and other activists such as Emma Goldman paved the way for subsequent generations of women to say when and if they would bear children. Coming on the heels of the suffragist movement that granted women the right to vote, this was a significant foundation for the coming "Women's Rights" movement, which in turn, created our current feminist advances. Without people like Margaret Sanger, reading this book would be illegal.

I read once that men sought to subjugate women because when they looked at each one, they saw the face of the Goddess they had scorned. When we honor our full empowerment, we reclaim the rejected Goddess and give her life on earth through our smile, through our love, and through our strength. Personally, I believe they were jealous that we could do such a cool thing and had to get their egos all mixed up with it.

One of the ways we honor our own inner Goddess is by taking full responsibility for our own sexuality. YOU decide with whom you will share yourself sexually and what you will and will not do sexually. Have sex deliberately and "on purpose" with tremendous focus and revel in the pleasure of it. If you are not in the mood, it does not happen. When it does happen, it is on your terms. Your needs, your orgasm, your pleasure, and your comfort are just as important as your partner's *every single time*. If you want to spend a session of lovemaking in which you only give and do not receive, do so with an air of reverence and power because you choose to give of yourself.

Take responsibility for your own contraception and do not rely on your partner to make those choices unless you are in a committed relationship and have an agreed contraceptive protocol. Never have a baby or give up a baby to fulfill the needs of another person (surrogacy being the exception).

Embrace your own sexual power and make your own rules. Honor the Goddess that you are.

CHAPTER 2 – SYMPTOMS OF PREGNANCY AND THE FIRST TRIMESTER (Up to 12 Weeks)

Signs and Symptoms of Pregnancy

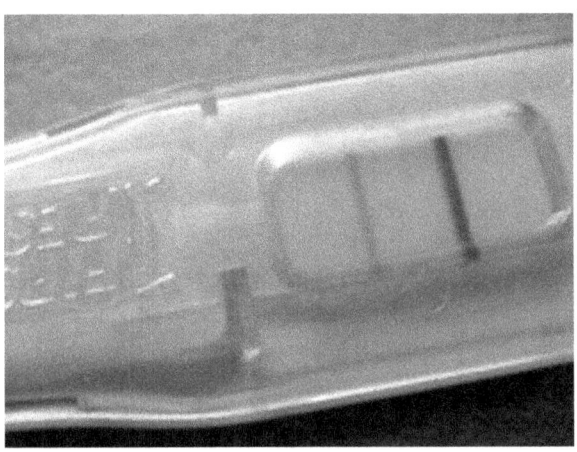

Just as every woman is different, every pregnancy is different even in the same woman. Some people have signs of pregnancy and some do not. Some people have different symptoms with different pregnancies. One would think that once a woman has been pregnant before, it would be easier for her to tell if she is pregnant again. This is not necessarily true since, as mentioned, each pregnancy tends to carry with it its own set of symptoms and characteristics.

In movies, television, and literature, often a woman learns she is pregnant when she drops into a faint for no apparent reason. Although that does occasionally happen due to increased blood volume and hormonal changes, other symptoms are far more common than fainting.

Missed Period: A woman will usually miss a period two weeks or so after conception. Sometimes, she may still have a light period while pregnant. There is also sometimes light bleeding at the time of implantation, which can happen just before the usual time of her period. Cramping may also occur with implantation. If a woman does not have regular periods, she may go for some time without realizing she is pregnant.

Chadwick's Sign: Approximately four to six weeks after conception, the cervix, labia, and vagina of a pregnant woman will turn a bluish, purplish color due to increased blood volume. This is more visible in a first pregnancy than in subsequent pregnancies.

Breast Changes: Even as early as one to two weeks after conception, a pregnant woman may have tenderness and slight swelling in her breasts. Since many women have this just prior the onset of their period, they may not register this as a symptom of pregnancy. The areolas will usually darken and enlarge slightly.

Extreme Fatigue: From a week after conception, women may begin to notice tremendous fatigue and sleepiness. This is likely one of the most common signs of pregnancy. The woman in her early pregnancy often wants to sleep all the time from total exhaustion. The body is changing gears and preparing to nourish two people instead of one and energy stores are depleted in doing so. A huge release of the hormone progesterone, increase in blood production, and lower blood sugar contribute to the extreme fatigue.

Nausea: Called "morning sickness" for its frequent appearance on wakening, this symptom usually manifests in the first two months after conception. Although "morning sickness" refers to nausea felt upon rising, it is common for nausea to occur throughout the day. Nausea can often be lessened by making certain the stomach is not empty for very long at a time. Eating crackers before getting out of bed can help absorb excess stomach acids before getting up for the day. Usually, this extreme nausea goes away by the twelfth week of pregnancy. Some women feel no nausea and some are very nauseated until they deliver the baby.

Most women who suffer from morning sickness are able to isolate specific foods that help or worsen the nausea. Heartburn is also common and some women find that eating a slice of bread or a few spoons of ice cream alleviates the discomfort. Most caregivers are not opposed to the use of an antacid.

Backaches: As soon as conception occurs, the uterus begins to gain weight from the extra lining and a slight swelling from the irritation of the implantation. This can put pressure on the ligaments that hold the uterus in place, causing minor back pain. Cramping at the time of implantation can also radiate into the back.

Headaches: From the point of fertilization onward, massive amounts of female hormones release in a complicated cocktail to support the pregnancy and protect the mother and baby. This spike in hormones can cause mild headaches or even migraines. This usually abates by twelve weeks when the body adjusts to the increased hormones.

Frequent Urination: Early in pregnancy, the swelling of the uterus pushes the bladder against the pubic bone, which causes pressure on the bladder and frequent urination.

Food Cravings or Aversions: Either of these conditions can begin in early pregnancy and last well into pregnancy. Food preferences may be extreme and often reflect a particular vitamin or mineral deficiency in the woman's body. Cravings for odd food combinations are also common, such as ice cream with tomatoes or pickles.

Vaginal Discharge: Hormonal changes affect the walls of the vagina shortly after pregnancy, causing them to begin to moisten and thicken. The pregnant mother may also experience a thin, milky-white discharge from the rapid increase in vaginal cell growth. There is typically no odor, burning or itching that accompanies this discharge.

Constipation: Progesterone, the hormone that causes fatigue in pregnant women, can also slow down intestine activity, resulting in constipation. An increase in water consumed, exercise, and eating plenty of high fiber foods can ease this discomfort.

Emotional shifts: The hormonal blast of early pregnancy often causes extreme emotional outbursts from anger to crying to fear to giddiness. This emotional instability can be challenging for both the pregnant mother and the people around her. It is very common for a pregnant woman to sob uncontrollably and have no idea why she is crying or to laugh at very inappropriate times.

Anatomy of the First Trimester

The **placenta** is a soft, porous organ about the size and shape of a pancake. It attaches to the wall of the uterus and acts as a transfer station for material between the mother and baby. Between the wall of the uterus and the placenta, there is a semi-permeable membrane that has perforations in it that are large enough to allow the material carried by blood cells through the membrane, but not the actual blood cells themselves, which are too large.

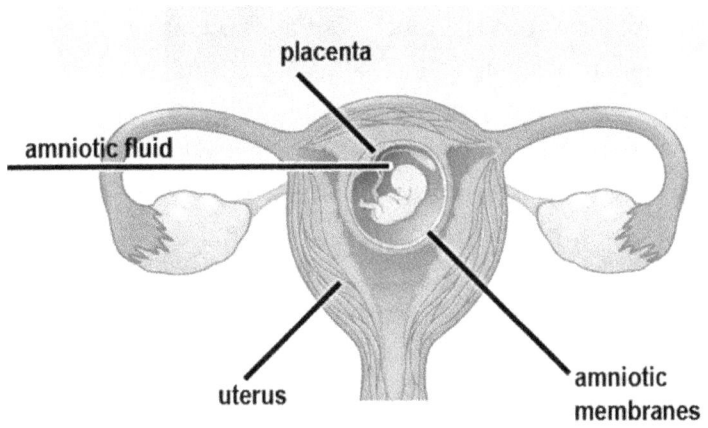

placenta

amniotic fluid

uterus

amniotic membranes

This allows the mother's bloodstream to transport nutrition, oxygen, and contaminants to the placenta and the baby to send carbon dioxide and body waste to the mother to release without the two bloodstreams ever mixing. The only time mixing of the bloodstreams occurs is when the placenta separates at birth and the semi-permeable membrane tears upon release. The placenta develops around the fourth week and begins to function around the tenth week. Prior to the tenth week, the uterine lining that would have been the mother's period nourishes the embryo.

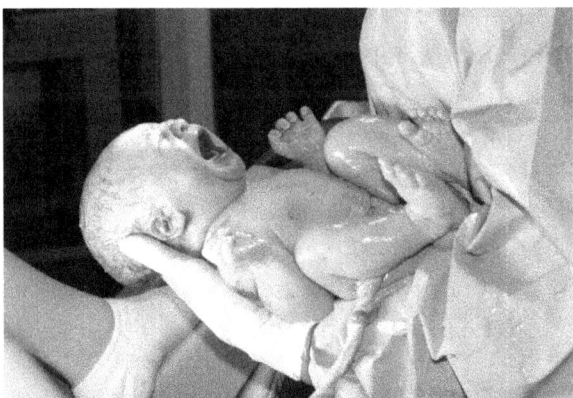

(A very angry) Newborn with an active umbilical cord

The **umbilical cord** is a tough cord approximately twelve to eighteen inches long and about as big around as a person's thumb. It is a bluish gray color when it is active, but when the baby is born and the cord is cut, it quickly begins to reduce in size and turn a pale white due to the loss of blood flow.

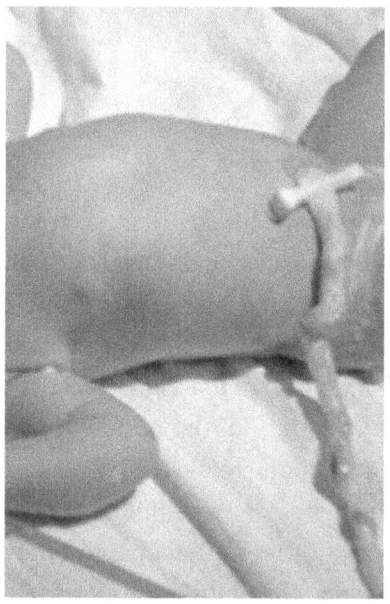

The cord is covered with a substance called "Wharton's Jelly" that, when exposed to air, begins to constrict and cut off blood flow between the baby and the placenta. You can see that the umbilical cord on the baby to the left is already beginning to turn white and constrict.

Prenatally, the umbilical cord connects roughly to the center of the placenta on one end and to the baby's navel on the other end. The navel is not closed prior to birth and for the first one to two weeks after birth.

The umbilical cord contains within it two arteries and a vein providing the circulatory process between the baby and the placenta. The umbilical cord exits the mother's body when the baby and the placenta are born.

To recap, all of the baby's nutrients (plus any contaminants in the mother's bloodstream) travel from the mother's bloodstream to the placenta and then to the baby by way of the umbilical cord. This also includes the baby's oxygen since it does not breathe in the uterus. Once the baby has processed all that it receives, it then passes all of its wastes back to the mother through the umbilical cord to the placenta.

Once the fetus's digestive system is able to function, the baby will swallow amniotic fluid, pass it through the digestive system, and urinate it out. This is not urine as we know it because the impurities of the body leave by way of the umbilical cord and placenta. It is merely funneling the fluid through the body to prime the digestive system for use after the baby is born.

Extending from all sides of the placenta to encompass the baby are the **amniotic membranes**. The membranes act as one membrane; however, there are actually two: the **amnion** and the **chorion.**

The function of the amniotic membranes is to hold in the amniotic fluid during the duration of the pregnancy and to provide a barrier against infection for the baby during pregnancy. The placenta, cord, and the amniotic membranes are what is referred to as "the afterbirth."

Seven to Eight Weeks After Conception

Almost immediately after a woman conceives, the cervix (the bottleneck opening of the uterus) begins to fill with thick mucus. This mucus remains in place until just prior to labor. This is called the "mucus plug" and is released when the mother's cervix begins to open during or just before labor. The mucus plug acts as a secondary protection against infection, blocking the cervix from any impurities that might be present in the vaginal canal. The amniotic membranes act as the primary barrier against infection and keep the baby safely enclosed until birth if the mucus plug is lost.

The **amniotic fluid** regulates the temperature around the baby so that there are no hot spots or cold spots. If the mother goes into an environment that is particularly hot or cold, the fluid around the baby will heat up or cool down gradually rather than all at once.

The fluid also acts as a cushion or shock absorber if the mother happens to bump into something with her belly or take a fall. If there is an accident of some kind, the baby is usually safe as long as the placenta remains intact and the amniotic membranes do not rupture.

Typical Lab Work and Testing

Most women take a home pregnancy test initially and then go to a doctor, midwife, or nurse practitioner for confirmation. Pregnancy tests, whether commercially available or through a medical professional, measure the amount of human chorionic gonadotropin (HCG) in a woman's bloodstream or urine. HCG is a hormone that sustains the pregnancy and tells body not to reject the fertilized egg as a foreign object. This hormone peaks and then drops by the twelfth week when the pregnancy becomes self-sustaining. Some medical professionals will use an ultrasound machine, also called a "sonogram," to confirm the pregnancy.

Early in the pregnancy, the sonogram is usually done with a vaginal probe rather than through the abdomen as is common later in the pregnancy. The sonogram bounces sound waves off of internal organs and then produces an image on a monitor of what is inside the body. This sonogram may be repeated at twenty weeks or later to attempt to determine the gender of the baby.

Initial Pregnancy Lab Work:

Blood Typing – This test determines your blood type, Rh type, and antibody factor. If your blood type is Rh negative, special monitoring of your blood may be necessary to check for Rh incompatibility.

Antibody Screen – detects unusual antibodies that may have arisen in a prior pregnancy or from a blood transfusion.

CBC (Complete Blood Count) – This test checks your blood to determine if you are anemic. Platelet levels are also assessed. These are necessary for coagulation.

Rubella Test (German Measles) – an antibody test to determine if you are protected from Rubella, which creates problems when contracted during pregnancy.

Syphilis Screening (RPR/VDRL) – tests for exposure to syphilis. If present, treatment can be initiated so that the fetus is not harmed.

Hepatitis B (HBSAG) – checks for infection with the Hepatitis B virus, which can be passed to an unborn child.

Glucose Screening – If an initial blood sugar level is high or borderline, more extensive testing may be ordered to monitor for Gestational Diabetes, a form of diabetes specific to pregnancy.

Hepatitis C – Hepatitis C is a viral infection of the liver. A simple blood test can be done to detect the infection.

HIV – test that checks for the AIDS virus. If you have HIV infection, you can be treated during pregnancy, which will reduce the chances of you passing the virus to your unborn child.

At the Time of the First Physical Examination:

Pap smear – checks for abnormal cervical cells.

Vaginal cultures - tests may be performed for vaginitis; candidia, gardnerella, gonorrhea, Chlamydia, and trichomonas.

Landmarks Specific to Early Pregnancy

If a woman does not miss a period or normally has irregular periods, she may not know she is pregnant until she reaches the second trimester and other symptoms begin to emerge.

A common feeling among women in early pregnancy is that the pregnancy was a dream or that it is not real. This is particularly true if they do not experience many of the previously listed symptoms.

Men often have a similar feeling of near-ambivalence that can extend until the baby is actually born. An old saying is, "A woman is a mother as soon as she conceives, but a man is a father when the baby he sees." Since women feels the baby on an ongoing basis, it is often more "real" to them. For men, it may not be real until they can see it. This can create friction between expectant couples, especially when the heightened emotions of the pregnant woman come into play.

The first trimester may be a time of confusion and fear if the pregnancy is unplanned. Decisions sometimes have to be made about whether to continue the pregnancy and consideration is given to life changes that will take place because of the pregnancy.

The determination of a due date is based on the date of the first day of the last menstrual period or the date of conception, if it is known. The typical pregnancy lasts forty weeks; however, most medical professionals consider babies born at thirty-eight to forty-two weeks to be "term" babies. Progressive caretakers do not use numbers, but rather the baby's physical condition to assess whether a baby is pre-term, term, or post-due. Babycenter.com offers a quick and easy due date calculator for a general idea of when a baby is likely to be born.

Most women will see their caregiver every four weeks until the twenty-eighth week.

A Word About Miscarriage

Miscarriages usually happen prior to the twelfth week of pregnancy. Women will sometimes miscarry and not realize they were pregnant, thinking they are merely having a late period that is heavy as a result. Educated estimates say that one pregnancy in four ends in a miscarriage and that the average woman who is sexually active will have approximately four miscarriages during her childbearing years.

The medical term for a miscarriage is a "spontaneous abortion" as opposed to an "elective abortion" or "therapeutic abortion" to end a pregnancy by choice.

It is rare for babies born before the twentieth week to be viable, but it does happen. Of those who live, profound birth defects are common. A baby who is born at twenty to thirty-six weeks and lives is called a premature birth. A baby born after the twentieth week who does not survive is said to be stillborn.

Prior to twelve weeks, the miscarriage will usually be "complete," meaning that all materials of the pregnancy leave the woman's body spontaneously. After twelve weeks, it is more common for the placenta to have difficulty separating. If this is the case, a "D&C" (dilation and curettage) is usually required to surgically remove any remaining pregnancy material from inside the uterus.

Miscarriage is an emotionally troubling experience that is rarely given the degree of attention needed. It is difficult for those around the mother to know how to grieve with her and for her and this results in damaging comments such as "It was probably for the best," or "You can always have more children" or "It wasn't even really a baby yet." One of the worst things a person can say is, "I understand" unless they are someone who has actually experienced a loss of pregnancy.

The best way to comfort a grieving woman who has suffered a miscarriage is to let her talk when she wants to do so and otherwise, to offer emotional support and comfort measures (not platitudes). It is also important to remember that the father of the baby may also be grieving and need attention. Often, emphasis is with the mother and her partner's feelings may be disregarded since they are often seen as a "support team." The partner usually feels the loss as significantly as does the mother and should also be considered.

The Spiritual Aspect of the First Trimester

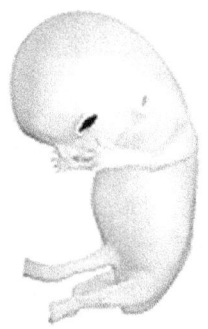

Whether your pregnancy comes as a surprise or was planned, the first semester is quite a roller coaster ride of emotions and body changes. For a good bit of her first trimester, the mother may not even yet know that she is pregnant and it can come as quite a surprise, as we all know, bringing with it stunned and varied emotions. These extreme emotional reactions and fluctuations may confuse the partner of a pregnant woman. They can happen even if this was an eagerly planned and anticipated pregnancy. Women will feel their power rise and fall as they adapt to their new body chemical levels and sensations. If a woman has miscarried before, this can be a scary time and she might resist bonding with the baby until she passes the point in her pregnancy where she suffered the loss before.

My husband has a theory with which I agree whole-heartedly that a baby's personality is affected by the energy that surrounds the parents at the time of conception. Of course, we have no clinical studies or reports to back this observation because it is merely that, an observation. Babies conceived in a peaceful and happy environment seem to have a friendlier and calmer disposition. Babies conceived in a stressed, frantic, or angry environment tend to be more high strung and irritable.

We believe this is due to the energy transference between mother and baby when the baby is going through its most formative time. Later in pregnancy, we can see babies respond to a mother's emotional state, becoming calm when she is calm and experiencing rapid heart tones and signs of stress when she is emotionally stressed. A mother-child bond that exists later in pregnancy could very well exist early in pregnancy.

The Alan Guttmacher Institute reports that in 2008, 51% of pregnancies were unintended and of those pregnancies, 40% ended in termination. This study also states that of single fathers involved in an unintended pregnancy, 10% did not know about the pregnancy until after the baby was born.

This means that the first part of a woman's pregnancy can be one of the most tumultuous times of her life and it is in those times that we often feel that we are divorced from God or The Goddess and that our lives are careening off course. Very little can be a game changer as a pregnancy can.

On the other hand, for those who are trying to become pregnant or are open to being so if not actively trying, this can be an exuberant and celebratory occasion. As I have said, each woman has her own experience, even pregnancy to pregnancy. Regardless, this is a time of tremendous change and deep spiritual contemplation.

Sometimes, a woman employs the power inherent in secrecy during this time. Many women do not make their pregnancy public knowledge until the pass that vital twelve-week point where miscarriage is less likely, especially if they have experienced losses before. Since a woman typically does not "show" during this time, her secret can be her own unless she is vomiting on a regular basis to the point that people fear she is dying.

Our interpersonal relationships are bound to be affected by each of our pregnancies and our plans for the future may shift, whether or not the pregnancy is intentional. In one of my relationships, my partner believed that my newly discovered and completely unexpected pregnancy would be the glue that brought us closer together. On the contrary, it was what convinced me that he was not the person I wanted my child to base its opinion of men upon, so I ended the relationship. Very little catalyzes change like a baby.

This is a prime time to get to know yourself, your motivations, and your deepest insecurities. If we buy into the premise that "everything happens for a reason" and has its place in the process of our lives, we have to consider how this pregnancy affects our trajectory and rearranges our plans. Pregnancy starkly defines where we are in the world and how suited we are or are not to parenthood. Ideally, we establish all of those things before we create situations in which pregnancy is a possible outcome; however, even having done so, pregnancy is a snap-focus for the reality of what was previously only an idea.

This can also be a stressful time if the pregnant mother is foregoing unhealthy habits in favor of her baby's health, such as giving up smoking, drinking, caffeine, or prescription medications that could be harmful. Not only does her body have to adjust to these changes, but her emotions have to regulate when those comfort measures and addiction responses are no longer available to her.

Use the first trimester of your pregnancy as a time of adaptation and flow. Your body is changing in remarkable ways and the chemicals that determine your mood and your body functions are in high flux. Be gentle and patient with yourself and try to avoid situations where you feel rushed or pressured. Meditate. Breathe. Pray. Surround yourself with lovely things and lovely environments. Bond with the people closest to you. Simplify, simplify, simplify. Let go of what no longer serves you and streamline your life so that it runs more efficiently and does not require as much input from you. Strip away extraneous obligations and declutter your output stream.

If you are spiritually open to the idea, try connecting into the Great Mother, the Mother Goddess, and feel her graciousness move through you, blessing your body and your baby. Ask for the ability to trust yourself, your choices, and your body. Release the pains, hurts, and offenses of the past and clear your slate for the coming weeks and months. Be completely present and in the moment of your life and your pregnancy. Really plug in and see what this pregnancy does and does not do for you. Find out what gifts it brings in addition to a baby. Think about what you want to create in your own life, just as you are creating life within.

Think about the incredible miracle of nature that is unfolding right there in your uterus. Cell division is occurring at such a phenomenal rate. Every day, a new physical feature or process develops further. Tap into that energy and let it merge into your own changes and share that incredible efficiency. Relax and let go, releasing your worries, your fears, and your insecurities to whatever power you consider holy and sacred. Be in one moment fully, then the next and the next. Be mindful, but do not be afraid to vision and drift from time to time. Your energy is very ethereal when you are newly pregnant as your spirit incorporates the new changes.

Take deep breaths and center on the movement of air into and out of your body. Imagine that the air is cleansing, clearing, and nourishing. Imagine that your air and your energy are blessing your baby and providing all it needs to grow and develop. Know that your body will do the same for you as well.

CHAPTER 3 – THE SECOND TRIMESTER (13-28 Weeks)

Landmarks Specific to the Second Trimester

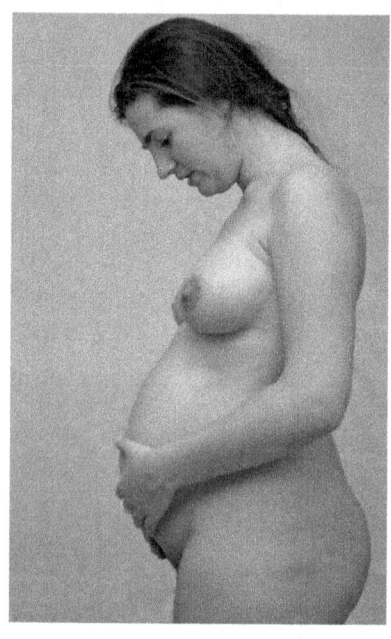

Compared to the excitement of the first trimester and the preparation for impending delivery that takes place in the third trimester, the second trimester is usually fairly mellow and uneventful.

Most women feel that the second trimester is the most comfortable time of their pregnancy and the "glow" common to pregnant women is usually present by now. The nausea and extreme fatigue are starting to abate by now and that definitely helps with the "glow" process. Many women report that during their second trimester, they feel incredibly healthy and energetic.

Breasts become fuller and firmer as prolactin begins to move through the ducts, priming them to produce colostrum in the last few weeks of pregnancy. There may be a darkening and enlarging of the nipples and areole. A friend of mine calls this time, "The arrival of the Titty Fairy."

By the end of the trimester, there is a definite roundness to the mother's belly as she begins to "show." How quickly a pregnancy is visible has everything to do with the mother's physical structure. Short women tend to show faster than tall women. Thinner women show faster than larger women. Some women go into maternity clothing before their pregnancy is readily apparent because their jeans will no longer close and shirts are now tight. Some opt to wear looser non-maternity clothing for most of the pregnancy.

The pregnant mother will usually begin to feel the baby move somewhere between sixteen and twenty weeks, earlier for moms who have been pregnant before because they are more familiar with the feeling. This is still several weeks before another person will be able to feel the baby's movements through her tummy, which usually happens around twenty-eight to thirty weeks. The mother may not at first realize what she is feeling since the movement of a small baby feels more like fluttering at first or just a tummy lurch.

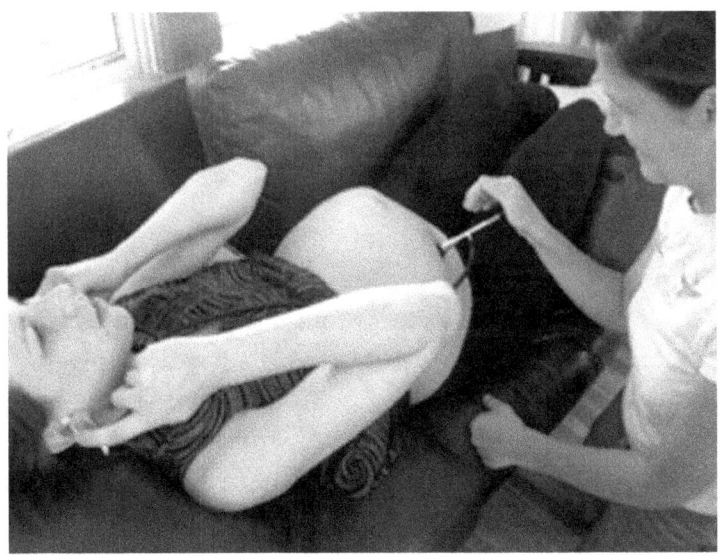

A midwife using a fetoscope to hear heart tones

At approximately twelve weeks, the health care providers begin to expect that they will hear heart tones using specialized instruments. One such instrument is a fetoscope, seen above.

The baby's heartbeat can also be detected using a "dopler" which usually has an amplified speaker that allows others in the room to hear the fetal heart tones:

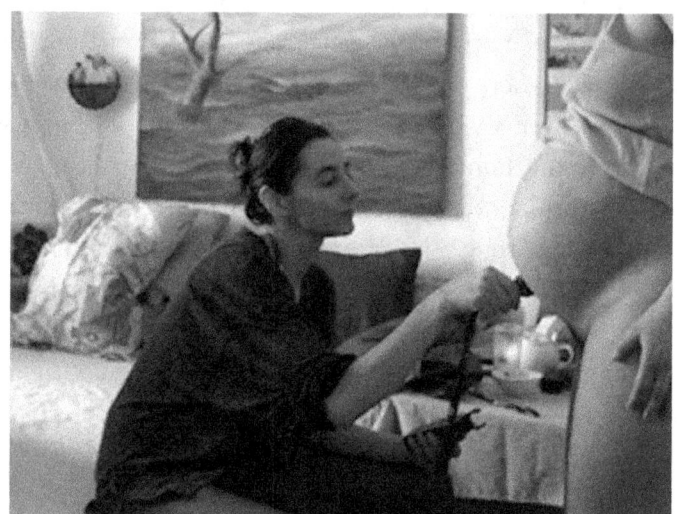

A midwife checks heart tones with a dopler

Normal heart rate for an unborn baby is 120-160 beats per minute. The heart rate slows as the baby grows. Some people believe the heart rate is one way to determine the gender of an unborn baby. As adults, the heart rate of a female is faster than the heart rate of a male, so the theory is that a fetal heart rate of 120-140 is a boy baby and 140-160 is a girl baby.

The frequent urination of the first trimester usually resolves because the uterus had grown large enough to pop up over the pubic bone, reducing the pressure on the bladder. Once the baby "drops" in the last few weeks of pregnancy, this frequent urination will return (with friends).

Routine prenatal exams usually begin with the second trimester. A typical prenatal exam will include a urinalysis to check for protein in the urine (a sign of pre-eclampsia – a condition related to blood pressure) and glucose in the urine (to check for high blood sugar). The pregnant woman's blood pressure will be checked and she will be weighed. The baby's heartbeat will be checked and the "fundal height" will be measured using a centimeter tape by placing end of the tape on the mother's pubic bone and measuring the top of the uterus, called the fundus. Interestingly, the height in centimeters usually equals the number of weeks she is pregnant:

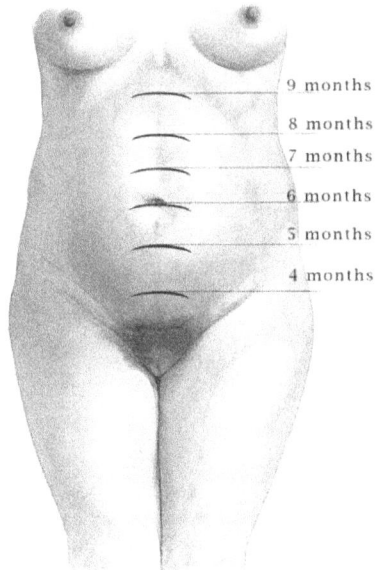

9 months
8 months
7 months
6 months
5 months
4 months

Usually around the twentieth week, an ultrasound/sonogram is performed to verify the expected delivery date, check for any obvious abnormalities, and possibly determine the gender of the baby. The quality of sonogram images available depends on the level of sophistication of the machinery used. Most facilities will print out a picture of the image for the parents.

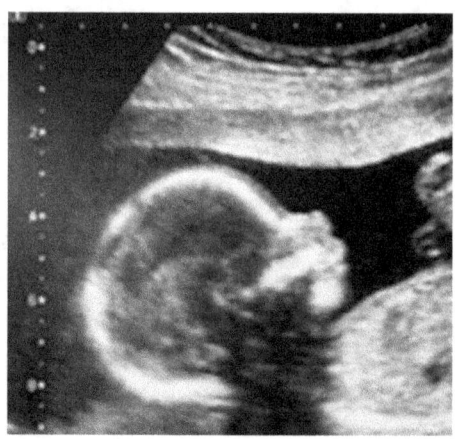
A typical ultrasound picture above.

This is the machine that takes the ultrasound pictures:

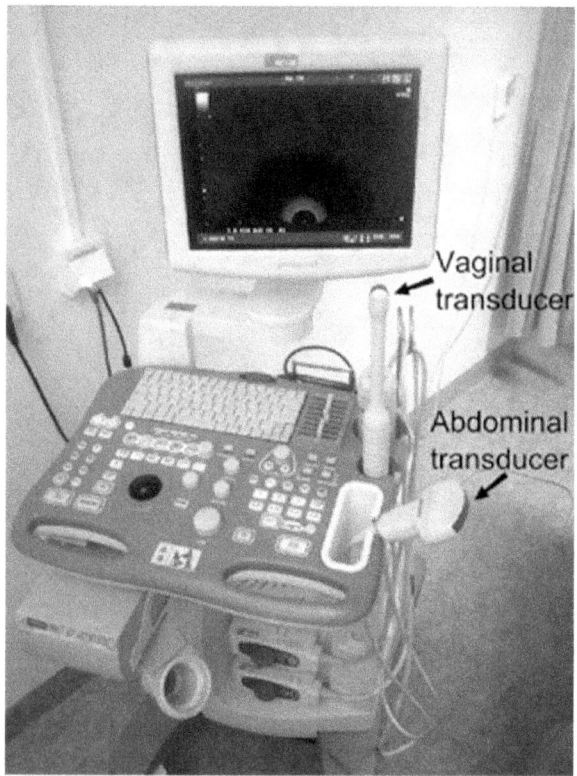

The picture of the baby, uterus, and other internal structures show up on the computer monitor screen. The technician will use either the abdominal transducer, which is rubbed over the mother's bare tummy with the use of conductive jelly (a lot like KY Jelly) or the vaginal transducer, which gets a condom looking protective sleeve over it and goes into her vagina.

This is what it looks like to get a prenatal ultrasound:

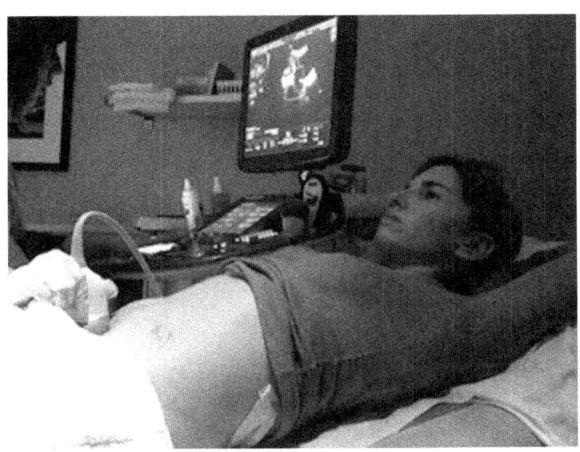

Possible Lab Work at 15-20 Weeks:

Alpha-Fetoprotein Testing – This is a genetic screening test administered in the critical window of fifteen to twenty weeks. The purpose is to screen for neural tube defects such as spinal bifida (the spinal cord is exposed) or hydrocephaly (water on the brain), as well as Down syndrome. The "AFT" has an unfortunate propensity for false positive results. A positive alpha-fetoprotein test opens the door for parents to have further genetic testing such as an amniocentesis in which a needle is inserted into the amniotic fluid through the mother's abdomen. A sample of the amniotic fluid is withdrawn for testing. Amniocentesis provides more definitive results and can diagnoses neural tube defects and Down syndrome, as well as determine lung maturity and the gender of the baby.

When an "amnio" is performed, the technician uses ultrasound images to make certain the needle enters into the amniotic sac away from where the baby is located. The amniotic membrane usually heals spontaneously from the small needle penetration. Even in our time of advanced medicine, there is still considerable risk involved in an amniocentesis.

Possible Lab Work at 28 Weeks:

Glucose Screening – If there is concern for the blood sugar levels of the pregnant mother, her caregiver may request various levels of testing at this time. This is to monitor for gestational diabetes, a form of diabetes that only manifests during pregnancy.

Rh Testing – If the mother tested as Rh negative during her initial screening, she will possibly have a follow up antibody screen. This will check for the development of antibodies against the Rh positive blood cells that may exist in the baby. If a mother's system detects Rh positive cells, it will develop antibodies that will attempt to destroy the Rh positive cells. Drugs such as "Rhogam" or "Rhophylac" keep the body for developing these antibodies. Medication for this condition is typically administered at twenty-eight weeks and again at thirty-six weeks. A mom's body will not usually develop antibodies during her first pregnancy as there needs to be an initial mixing of bloodstreams for the mother's body to know about the positive antibodies. Unfortunately, not all mothers are truthful about the number of pregnancies they have experienced (an abortion, for instance) or may not be aware they miscarried, resulting in mixed bloodstreams. It is also possible to develop antibodies after a blood transfusion. This is why all mothers who are Rh negative are treated.

CBC – Complete blood test to check for anemia.

GBS – The mother may possibly be cultured for strep B.

The Spiritual Aspect of the Second Trimester

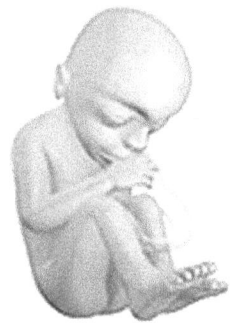

By the second trimester, most women have become more peaceful about their pregnancy, whether it is coming down off the initial rush of excitement or reconciling the reality of the pregnancy in their own mind. After the twelfth week, in most locations of the United States, the mother is past the point of legally terminating the pregnancy, so without major decisions to make and with the prospect of labor still far in the future, she is free to relax and enjoy being pregnant. There is not usually a great deal of discomfort yet, so she probably sleeps well and has a healthy appetite and a good energy supply.

The greatest change during the second trimester is that of visibility. By twenty to twenty-four weeks, the pregnancy usually becomes obvious. The mother begins to feel active movement from the baby that she recognizes and these two factors make the pregnancy much more "real" for her. It is easier to bond to the baby when she feels movement on a regular basis. By the end of this trimester, her partner and/or loved ones can also usually feel the baby move through her belly. This causes excitement to grow around her. Often loved ones will fawn over the pregnant woman, giving her attention, which can be gratifying. This is her time to shine.

Drifting between the discomforts of the last weeks of pregnancy and the hormonal and digestive disruptions of early pregnancy, this is likely the most comfortable the mother will be for the entire pregnancy.

Hormones, specifically progesterone, relaxin, and prolactin, are flowing at this time and generate a sense of well-being and peacefulness. This is a wonderful time to use those good feelings to connect in with the Divine and enjoy sacred space. Do not be surprised if your baby becomes very active when you meditate. Not only are you breathing deeply and increasing the blood oxygen supply, but you are also easing toward Delta wave activity, which is when your vibratory force is closest to that of the baby.

It can be especially potent to relax, meditate, and tune into your baby, sending it messages of welcome, of comfort, of love, and of acceptance. Gently massage your tummy over your uterus and imagine the energy from your hand reaching out to your baby. In your mind's eye, see your baby reaching back to you.

CHAPTER 4 – THE THIRD TRIMESTER (28 Weeks - Birth)

Landmarks Specific to the Third Trimester

As the last month of pregnancy nears, the pregnant mother usually becomes increasingly uncomfortable from the weight of the baby and from her own excess weight from food stores and water retention. Average weight gain for a healthy pregnancy is between twenty and forty pounds. Most of that weight is gained in the last trimester. The amount of weight a woman will gain with her pregnancy is extremely individual. As the baby grows bigger and the woman's uterus stretches, the pregnant mother may begin to feel ungainly and clumsy.

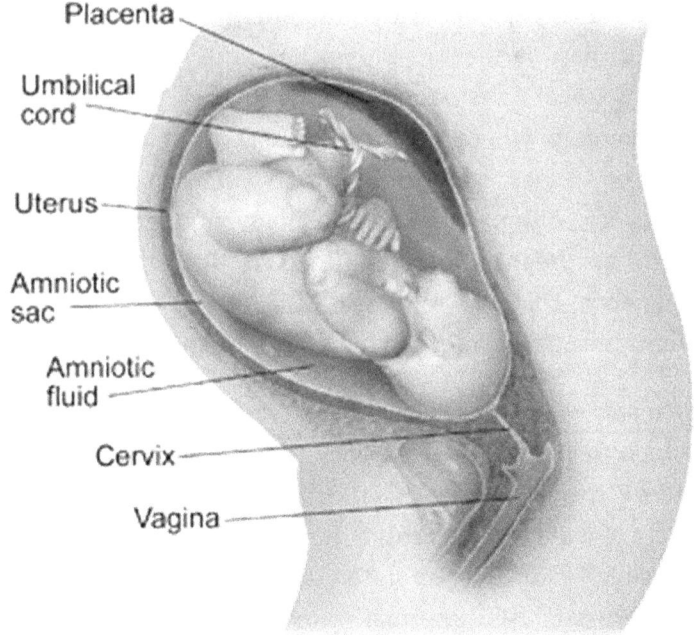

Internal anatomy at 34 weeks

Sometime around twenty-eight to thirty-two weeks is when most pregnant women begin attending prepared childbirth classes to educate themselves about the birth process, routine hospital procedures for their local area, and pain relief measures.

Stretch marks may appear on the skin of the breasts, belly, or hips. Stretch marks are a matter of genetic predisposition in a pregnant woman with normal weight gain. Excessive weight gain nearly always produces stretch marks. Creams and lotions help to make the belly, thigh, hip, and breast skin suppler, but none is guaranteed to prevent stretch marks.

If the mother lives with her partner, the partner may begin to have **sympathy symptoms** and experience some of the same sensations and discomfort as the pregnant mom. This can cause feelings of frustration in the pregnant woman as it feels her partner is interjecting into her experience beyond what she appreciates. This is a very true phenomenon where a woman's male partner will have lower backaches, nausea, and other symptoms common to pregnancy. Although we should be sympathetic since we often, as pregnant woman, tend to have those same experiences, it tends to instead cause us to stare at them intently and say comforting things like, "Really? *Really?!*"

Pregnant women usually have **strange dreams**. This happens all through pregnancy, but is especially typical toward the end of pregnancy. Many pregnant women dream of water, in the form of flowing water or large bodies of water. Women also often dream of the labor and delivery, not just in normal terms, but also with strange outcomes, such as giving birth to a chimp, the baby having no umbilical cord, or the baby being born as a toddler or adult.

Hormones released in late pregnancy may cause **darkening of the linea negra** (the vertical belly button line) and the nipples. The **belly button may invert** from internal pressure. Both of these changes will go away after the pregnancy is over.

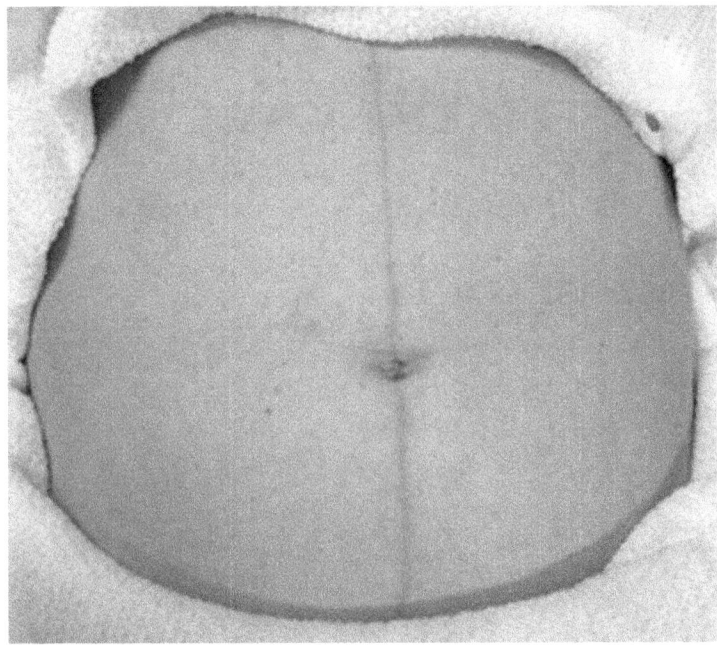

Linea negra. An OB/GYN doc once told me that it was proof positive that God intended women to have cesarean sections because he put the incision pattern right on their bellies. (Yes, roll your eyes here)

The same hormonal changes that darken the belly button line and the nipple can also cause the "**mask of pregnancy**," which is a darkening of the skin pigmentation around the eyes or on the cheeks and forehead.

The **uterosacral ligament** stretches from the lower back of the uterus to the sacrum. As the uterus grows heavy, it tips forward and puts stress on this ligament, which can cause lower back pain.

As it tips forward, the uterus rotates very slightly, which puts pressure on the **round ligaments**, usually on one side of the body. The round ligaments attach to the uterus on each side, halfway up the body of the uterus. They then join into the ligature of the pelvic floor. When the uterus turns slightly, one ligament is stretched more than the other. This can cause sharp, shooting pains in the lower abdomen just above where the leg joins the torso or midway up the abdomen in front of the ribs. This pain can be reduced by lying down on the side that hurts, which causes gravity to pull the uterus down slightly and lessen the tension on the ligament. Round ligament pains usually occur with an "over reach" or an abrupt torso turn.

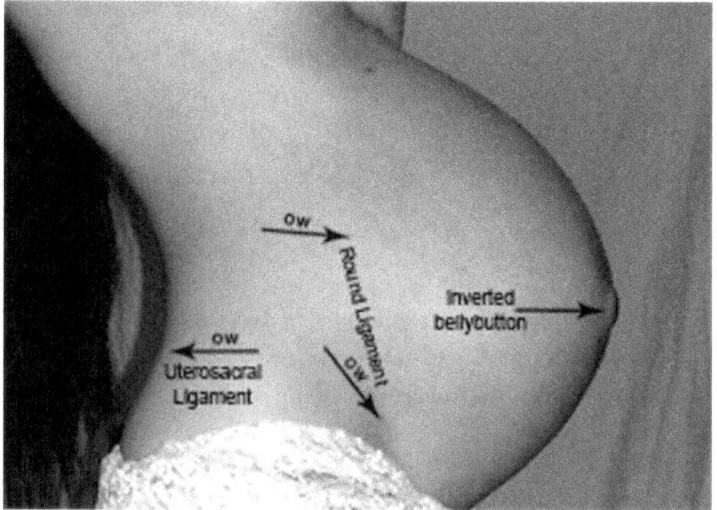

This beautiful pregnant belly photo is graciously shared by
Pyrosaint-Stoxon Deviant Art.
http://www.deviantart.com/art/Pregnancy-Misc-24-122611784

The uterus will stretch to approximately sixty times its normal size during a routine pregnancy. The uterus does have a maximum ability to stretch and one theory says that once the maximum stretch is reached, hormones will usually be released to cause the woman to go into labor.

This is why women carrying multiple babies often go into labor early. It is extremely rare for a uterus to rupture from pregnancy.

Relaxin, a hormone released by the placenta itself, causes the fibrocartilage in the pelvis and throughout the body to soften. This is particularly noticeable in the hips, near the pubic bone and on each side of the sacrum and results in painful **"creaking" sensations**, particularly when the pregnant woman has long periods of exercise (walking, for instance) or is sitting still in one position for a long time.

At this point in their pregnancies, women often become frustrated by the **liberties taken by others to touch their pregnant belly.** One would not usually touch the belly of a non-pregnant person, so this is actually quite rude. Women should be encouraged to ask others to respect their physical boundaries (or else, lean over and touch their belly right back). A theory is that this occurs once the pregnant belly has sufficiently grown to extend beyond the "personal space bubble" of the pregnant woman to become public domain. Saying "No touching, please" or gently removing their hands from the belly usually gets the point across.

Relaxin also causes the intestines to slow down even more and become sluggish, which can result in **constipation**. Many women fear pushing for a bowel movement when the baby's head is low. If the cervix is not open, the baby will not emerge. Eating plenty of fiber and drinking ample water is particularly essential at this time to combat constipation.

Additionally, Relaxin causes the tissues of the brain to "relax" and creates a condition known as "**pregnant brain**." Pregnant women may become foggy and disoriented at times, may use the wrong words in sentences, and temporarily forget basic concepts (like "driving"). This condition leaves immediately following birth. There is an overall sense of fogginess and disconnection that tends to show up later in the last trimester so that many pregnant women do not seem completely plugged into the "real" world. Don't worry. She will be back.

Indigestion may return as the growing baby begins to put pressure on the stomach. This is usually temporarily relieved when the baby "drops" further into the pelvis.

Feet, legs and hands may begin to swell due to fluid retention and poor leg circulation. This is particularly common in women who sit at a desk or in a car for long periods. It also tends to be worse during warm/hot weather.

Closer to time for delivery, the mother may notice a **milky or crusty discharge from her nipples** as the prolactin begins to activate her milk duct system. Breasts may again become sore as the milk ducts begin to enlarge and colostrums, the forerunner of breast milk, starts to push through the ducts.

As the uterus pushes further up into the lungs, many women – particularly those who are short-waisted – may experience **shortness of breath**. This is lessened when the uterus shifts in the last two to four weeks of pregnancy and descends further into the pelvis.

Sexual partners may worry during this trimester or even before about hurting the baby through intercourse. Although alternate positions may be desired for the mother's comfort, unless the prenatal caregiver orders otherwise, sexual activity may continue for as long as the mother feels comfortable. The baby will not make contact with the sexual partner since the baby is surrounded by the membranes and uterus. Babies are not judgey about getting poked in the head through the uterus a bit and do not have the mature thoughts that formulate into, "I'll BET they're having SEX!"

Heartburn and nausea may return as digestion slows in preparation for birth and the stomach is compressed by the uterus.

Spider veins, varicose veins, and hemorrhoids may result from poor circulation and increased blood supply.

The uterus becomes very heavy and puts tremendous pressure onto the bladder causing **frequent urination**. Pregnant women may need to urinate several times an hour and wake up through the night to pee.

Vaginal discharge increases in the last two to four weeks of pregnancy. This discharge assists the relaxin in softening the vaginal tissues in preparation for birth.

Emotional highs and lows are common during the last weeks of pregnancy from the tension of discomfort, interrupted sleep, and the impending birth as well as from hormonal shifts.

The pregnant mother may have **shooting pains in her cervix** from the pressure of the baby's head. These may be offset by having the mother get into a knee chest position that transfers the weight of the baby upwards by gravity. She should kneel with pillows between her uterus and her breasts, elbows and upper body on the floor or bed and butt in the air higher than the chest.

During the last few weeks of pregnancy, the cervix becomes particularly blood-rich with thousands of tiny capillaries overfilled. **Mild bleeding** from capillary rupture is extremely common at this time following a vaginal exam or sexual activity. Bright red bleeding or excessive bleeding, even as heavy as a normal period, should be reported to the woman's caregiver. Only occasional spotting is normal.

Braxton-Hicks contractions are preliminary contractions that exercise the uterine muscles in preparation for labor. The uterus contracts all through pregnancy, but becomes more noticeable as the baby grows. Sometimes, these contractions become sufficiently uncomfortable as to convince the mother that she is actually in labor. This is called "false labor" and is seen much more often in women who have delivered a baby before.

False labor can start and stop. It can actually create changes in the cervix toward birth progress; however, these contractions are usually irregular and fairly mild. False labor will be covered in more detail in the Chapter 5.

Prenatal exams typically change from every month to every two weeks at the twenty-eight week point and every week at the thirty-six week point.

Lab & Diagnostic Tests at 36 Weeks and Beyond

Depending on the caregiver, some of the previous lab tests may be repeated for verification.

If the mother is still pregnant at forty weeks, weekly tests may be performed to keep track of the baby's well being. One of them is a "**non-stress test**" in which the baby's heart rate is measured while it moves. This helps to determine if the baby is receiving enough oxygen.

As the placenta ages beyond its lifespan, the edges begin to calcify, which can reduce the oxygen flow to the baby. This reduction in oxygen is reflected in reduced movement and lowered heart tones.

The pregnant mother's blood pressure is carefully monitored for any signs of pre-eclampsia/toxemia, which is a blood pressure related condition of pregnancy.

The Last 2-4 Weeks of Pregnancy

In the last two to four weeks of pregnancy, many women will experience the following symptoms in various configurations. None are universal; a woman may have some, none, or all of these:

Night Restlessness – A popular theory states that the hormone prolactin, which stimulates the milk ducts to prepare for lactation, also puts the pregnant mother *on the same sleep schedule as her baby* in order to align her circadian rhythms with her baby's sleep schedule. Many pregnant women notice that when they are up for no reason in the middle of the night, the baby starts kicking almost immediately after they wake up. They will often presume the baby kicked and that is what woke them up when, in fact, the prolactin woke them up because the baby was about to wake up. If there is a recurring time when the pregnant woman wakes up on a regular basis, often that be when the baby will want its night feeding after birth. Babies tend to keep the same sleep schedule out of the uterus as they did in the uterus.

Lightening or "Dropping" - During the last month or so of pregnancy, the heavy uterus begins to sink into the pelvic cavity. This is not just the baby moving downward, but the uterus with the baby inside. Still, the usual comment is "the baby has dropped." For most people, lightening is a gradual process that occurs over several days.

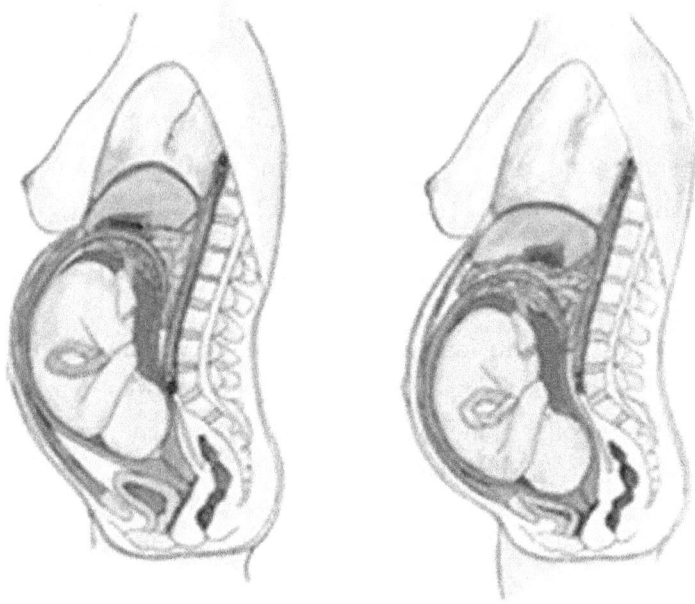

Lightening

Once lightening has occurred, the pressure on the bladder and pubic bone increases tremendously, but pressure on the lungs and stomach is reduced.

When the baby's head descends past the pubic bone and into the pelvic inlet, the baby's head is "**engaged**." The observable changes after a baby drops, as well as physical changes the mother feels, are more pronounced in women who are long-waisted. In women who have short torsos, there is not a lot of room for the baby to make a significant shift.

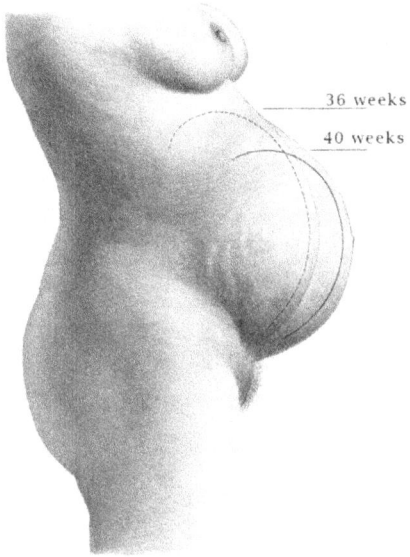

36 weeks

40 weeks

"Dropping" is often portrayed in movies and television as a sudden event that occurs overnight or in a matter of minutes. Typically, it happens over several days' time.

The degree to which the baby's head or other presenting part engages into the pelvis is measured in centimeters in relation to two bony protrusions on the woman's pelvis called the ischial spines. These are your "sit bones" that you feel when you sit upright on a hard surface and feel your butt bones touching the floor.

The arrows in the next illustration point to the ischial spines, which can be easily felt during a vaginal exam. The system of measurement of the degree of engagement is called "station." When the baby's head is even with the ischial spines, it is said to be at "0 station." One centimeter above the ischial spines is -1 station. Two centimeters above the ischial spines is -2 station and so on. At -4 station, the baby's head is free-floating even with the pubic bone and is not yet engaged.

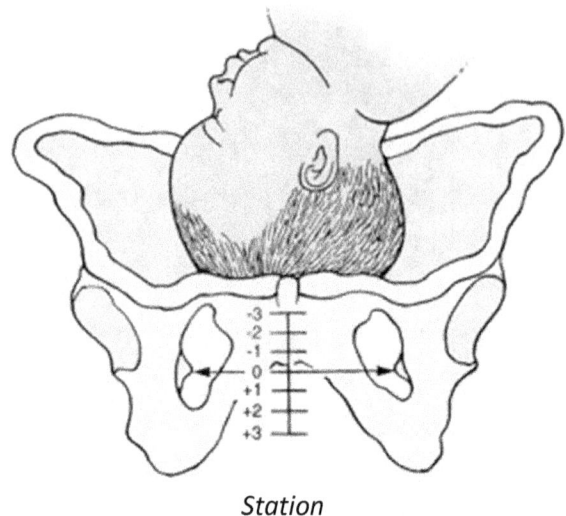

Station

The baby does not usually enter the plus stations until the mother is fully dilated and pushing. The baby will move further down during the contraction and when the contraction goes away, will slip back slightly, so the progression is something like two steps forward and one or one and a half steps back. This allows for a gentle and gradual pushing away of the vaginal walls. When the baby is at +4, the head is said to be crowning and passes under the pubic archway. At that point, it will no longer slip back.

Nesting – After weeks of lethargy and fogginess, many women feel a rush of energy in the last forty-eight hours or so before birth. This can be a general feeling of well being or a focused effort to complete tasks before the baby arrives. Pregnant women should be discouraged from overdoing so they are not exhausted when labor hits.

Release of the Mucus Plug – As the cervix starts to slowly open, often before the onset of actual labor through the efforts of the practice Braxton-Hicks contractions, the mucous plug begins to slip away. It is heavy, congealed mucus with blood tinged throughout from the capillaries that ruptured in the cervix as it releases.

Mild Diarrhea – Shortly before labor begins, many women experience diarrhea that helps to clear out the lower bowel in preparation for birth. If cramps accompany the diarrhea, a woman might mistake the cramping intestinal pain for labor. It is important to remember the pain from labor contractions will come and go. Intestinal cramping tends to be steady.

The Spiritual Aspect of the Third Trimester

The foggy, otherworldly feeling of the last four weeks of pregnancy in particular automatically lends itself to spiritual connection and it is a good time to capitalize on that connection to program yourself for an easy and healthy birth. Your brain is far more susceptible to suggestion during this time and during meditation, it can be very productive to visualize a safe and happy birth, as well as repeating affirmations: "I have all I need for a safe and happy birth." "My baby and I are blessed and happy." "My birth process is smooth, healthy, and uncomplicated."

Sleep as much as possible because physical discomforts often disrupt your normal sleep patterns and you will need to allow greater opportunity for restorative sleep. Continue to move, but do not over-exert yourself. Flex and stretch your muscles as you can, feeling the blood flow move through them and nourish them. Drink plenty of water and imagine that it is bringing a vital cleansing to your internal processes and to your baby. Be mindful of what you eat. Most pregnant women find that eating five or six small meals through the day is more comfortable than three large ones because of the pressure the uterus places on the stomach and the slowing down of digestion. Lungs and stomach are both able to hold approximately one quarter of their normal capacity in the last four weeks of pregnancy. Choose your foods wisely and give your body and your baby a variety of colorful, healthy foods.

Protect yourself from negative influences at this time because, as mentioned before, your mind is very susceptible to suggestion. As much as possible, keep your immediate environment and influences positive, encouraging, uplifting, and most of all *emotionally safe*. Many pregnant women feel a little frayed and raw at this time as the discomforts of late pregnancy and lack of solid sleep take hold. This is especially a time to be gentle with yourself and to feel what you feel; letting it wash over you, honoring it, and releasing it. During the last weeks of pregnancies, working mothers often begin to gear down, perhaps even beginning maternity leave.

Like all of the pregnancy process, each woman has her own experience during the last weeks of pregnancy. Your support team should work aggressively to keep you comfortable and to be particularly patient with you if you get grumpy, bitchy, or spacey. You will probably need both hugs and time alone, so the people around you should chart their course carefully and tread lightly. You should pay close attention to your own needs and honor them.

Since you are usually half between the worlds anyway, this continues to be a great time to meditate and work on positive affirmations for the birth process. Tune into your baby, who is growing by leaps and bounds now and, in fact, it is likely you feel your baby leaping and bounding in your belly until the last few days of pregnancy, when movement generally slows down due to lack of space for mobility. Anytime you go more than twenty-four hours without feeling your baby move, you should contact your health care provider. Usually, the baby is fine and the mother has simply become so accustomed to the baby's movements that she does not notice them as much.

Just keep dancing between the worlds, sweetheart. You are doing great. Focus on the necessary actions as best as you can and let the rest go. You are incubating and the world should stop for you. Sadly, that is rarely the case. There are reasons why we used to go into "confinement" at the end of pregnancy and shun the world except for our support system. In our modern life, however, that is typically not how it goes.

Be sure and make quiet time for yourself during the last part of your pregnancy for grounding, meditation, deep breathing, and active relaxation, which is relaxing when you are *not* sleeping, going through your entire body tensing and then fully releasing muscle groups until you kind of melt into the floor.

Learn what your body feels like tensed and relaxed. Have your partner gently touch your body as you relax into their hands so they can see and feel what your body is like both relaxed and tense.

Tense your muscles and have your partner hold that muscle, then relax into the pressure of your partner's hands. Learning to relax to touch is a very valuable tool in case sounds bother you during labor. Have your partner say, "Relax your ___" very softly. Learning to relax to voice suggestions is helpful if you find that being touched in labor is distracting to you. By training with both touch and voice, you will learn to respond automatically to either prompt in labor because they will both be familiar to you.

Feel the energy of the tension from your contracted muscle (arm, leg, hand, shoulders, etc) transfer into your partner's hands. Relax the muscle fully and completely into their hands. Do this all through the body, starting with your forehead, scrunching up your brow, and then to your jaw, your shoulders, all the way down to curling and releasing your toes.

Pay attention to how your body uses energy when it contracts and releases. Visualize pure, white light filling your body and blessing it with health, comfort, and positive energy.

As your partner strokes your body to help you relax, have them visualize healthy, vital energy moving from their hands into your body as you visualize the same thing.

CHAPTER 5 – EARLY LABOR

The uterus is comprised primarily of strong muscle tissue. During a labor contraction, it exerts a force of approximately forty-three pounds per square inch. The lateral muscles all around the sides of the uterus are in a figure 8 configuration. When the muscles contract, the result is that the fundus pushes onto the butt of the baby while the cervix is pulled back against the head with the uterine musculature pulling toward the middle. When these uterine contractions become regular and begin to cause changes in the ripened cervix, they are what some people call "labor pains."

During a contraction, the woman's abdomen, which is nearly all uterus at this point, will pull up and push outward, becoming very rigid. It will then relax when the contraction is over. Contrary to public opinion, labor is not nonstop pain. Contractions are intermittent, coming and going usually for hours, intensifying toward the end.

The effect of true labor contractions on the cervix is a process called **effacement** and **dilation** or **dilatation.** Effacement is the thinning and shortening of the cervix as it pulls up closer to the baby's head. The cervix starts out long and thick like a bottleneck. By the time early labor is over and active labor begins, it is thin and flat against the baby's head and feels like the webbing between your thumb and forefinger. Effacement is measured in percentages. A full, long, thick cervix is 0% effaced. A completely thin cervix that is does not extend downward and is completely flat against the baby's head is 100% effaced. Effacement occurs almost exclusively in early labor. Where does the cervix "go" when it effaces? It is incorporated up into the lower segment of the uterus.

Dilation is the actual opening up of the cervical os. The completion of the effacement process causes the full power of the contractions to go the dilation process. Since the cervix is now very thin, there is less of it to absorb the strength of the contraction and the dilation begins to occur much faster, which is what accelerates active labor. Dilation is measured in centimeters, the metric measurement. When the cervix is approximately ten centimeters dilated, it has receded sufficiently past the baby's head that the mother can begin to push out the baby. The process of effacement and dilation make up **the first stage of labor**. Effacement and dilation may ONLY be effectively determined through an internal vaginal exam by an experienced birth attendant.

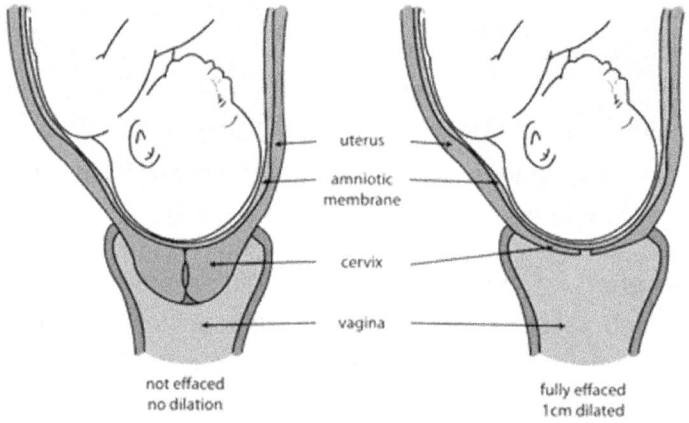

uterus

amniotic membrane

cervix

vagina

not effaced
no dilation

fully effaced
1cm dilated

Effacement in early labor

There are three phases of the first stage of labor: preliminary phase (early labor), active labor, and transition.

The preliminary phase or early labor, is the longest phase of the first stage of labor. It can last anywhere from hours to even days. Often, false labor and preliminary phase will blend so that it becomes difficult to ascertain when labor actually began.

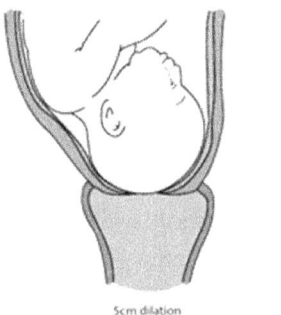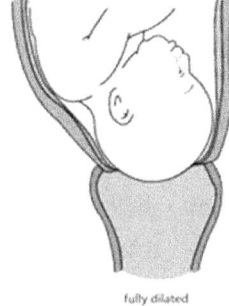

5cm dilation

fully dilated
at 10cm

Dilatation in active labor

Contractions are mild in preliminary phase, but may be strong enough to be uncomfortable and keep the mom awake. Contractions generally start out around twenty to thirty minutes apart and last from thirty to sixty seconds. This means that the mother has some time between contractions when she is not in pain and can function normally. She may become tired from a prolonged period of early labor or false labor. Exhaustion may cause the mother to perceive that the contractions are more painful than they actually are. Many women feel the unfamiliar sensation of a labor contraction and automatically interpret it as pain because they expect to feel pain.

The laboring mother should work to remain as relaxed as possible throughout her contractions. She should not begin her patterned breathing techniques (see Appendix 1) until she begins to have discomfort with her contractions strong enough to keep her from walking, talking, laughing, or finishing a sentence. Starting breathing techniques before they are needed can result in burnout very quickly since she may be doing them for a long time.

It is important that those around the laboring mom keep her centered and distracted during the labor process. If she focuses only on the contractions and the discomfort, her pain will increase. If early labor is suspected, she should be encouraged to eat very lightly to keep her strength up, sleep if she can at all, and if she cannot sleep, to walk around to try to speed up the labor. The effect of gravity combined with the movement of walking can intensify labor. Nipple and/or clitoral stimulation will also speed up labor since the same hormone that causes uterine contractions is released when a woman breastfeeds and when she is sexually aroused.

As labor starts, the digestive system begins to shut down to accommodate the tremendous energy required for childbirth. For this reason, the laboring mother should not eat heavy meals that are difficult to digest. In fact, she may find that her appetite goes away while she is in labor.

It is fine for a laboring woman to take a relaxing, warm bath as long as her amniotic membranes have yet not ruptured. She should be aware that while she is in the buoyancy of the warm water, the discomfort of her contractions will lessened. Immersion in warm water is a wonderful pain relief measure for labor.

This does mean, however, that her labor could progress further than she thinks it has while she is in the tub. Someone should always be with her, at least within voice range, if she is taking a bath in case she attempts to get out and finds she is in stronger labor than she thought.

As early labor progresses, the mucus plug loss and capillary rupture may continue, releasing more as effacement and dilation occur. The release of the mucous plug is a process that can happen over time, in either false labor or early labor.

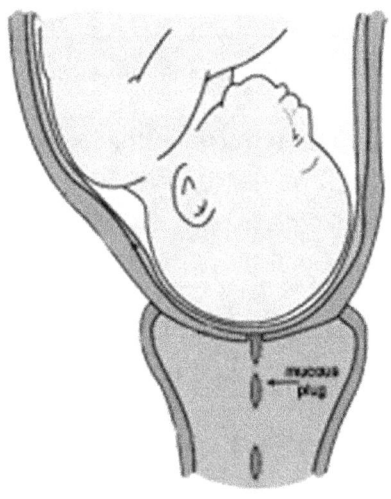

Mucous Plug Release

By the end of this phase, contractions are usually around **three to five minutes apart** and lasting **forty-five to sixty seconds**. **Effacement usually completes** and **dilation** is usually up to approximately **four to five centimeters** in this phase. Labor may stall out at around four to five centimeters while the effacement process completes. After effacement completes, dilation usually begins to progress rapidly.

True Labor VS False Labor

Determining the difference between true labor and false labor is a tricky task for anyone, even professionals. The issue is that there are no real absolutes, even though we can say what "generally" happens:

True labor contractions become progressively longer, stronger, and closer together and begin to set up a predictable pattern (every four minutes, for instance), with only a few seconds of variance. Both early labor and false labor can be very erratic, but true labor will usually begin to establish a set pattern with intervals between growing shorter and contractions growing longer and more intense.

Some women have contractions that do not settle into a pattern until they are well into active labor, so watch for other signs as well. This is particularly true for women who have previously given birth.

Some spotting may occur with true labor from capillary rupture as the cervix dilates.

Please note that it is common for a woman to go into true labor already three to four centimeters dilated and partially effaced from the effect of Braxton Hicks contractions.

Pay attention for the preliminary signs of oncoming labor covered in the last chapter such as nesting, mucus plug release, increased Braxton-Hicks contractions, mild diarrhea, and night restlessness.

Rupture of the Membranes

At some point during the labor process, the amniotic membranes will likely rupture, but it will usually not occur until a contraction of sufficient strength stresses the membranes beyond their capacity. Only ten to fifteen percent of laboring women have their membranes rupture before active labor begins. Sometimes, the membranes never spontaneously rupture and as the mother pushes, the membranes will bulge out of the cervix in front of the baby's head. Many birth attendants will leave the membranes intact for as long as possible to buffer the baby from the intense pressure of the contractions. If the labor begins to stall out, rupturing the membranes will speed things up because the hard head of the baby will then descend against the pelvis rather than the spongier membranes and fluid. If the membranes do not rupture, the attendant will sometimes pinch them as the mother pushes to break them.

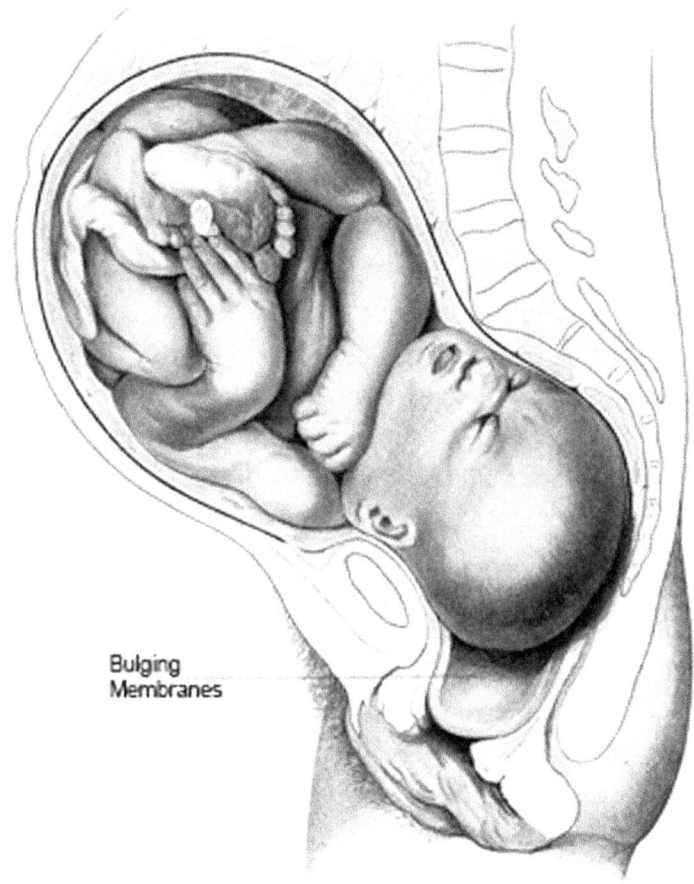

Bulging
Membranes

Another fallacy promoted by television and movies is that labor begins very suddenly and with a huge wave of pain. It is rare that labor begins with intense pain. More often, it is hours of "Is this it? I'm not sure if this is it. Is this it?"

Yet another misperception that is fueled by the entertainment industry is that you can tell how far a woman has progressed in labor by lifting her skirt and looking at her vagina. Unless she is completely dilated and the baby's head is on the way out, there is no way you can tell how far advanced her labor is by looking at a woman's vagina. The *cervix,* which is inside her body, not the vagina responds to the contractions of the uterus. The only way to determine the progress of labor is to perform a vaginal exam and feel the cervix in relationship to the baby's head and the baby's head in relation to the ischial spines.

Amniotic fluid is very warm and clear. There is about a liter of fluid in the uterus. The amniotic membranes will continue to produce amniotic fluid until the placenta is born following the baby's birth, so there is no such thing as the old wives' tale of a "dry" birth. Even after the membranes rupture and the fluid is released, the mother will continue to leak amniotic fluid from the vagina until the baby and the placenta is born.

Pockets of amniotic fluid may become trapped behind parts of the baby and release as the baby moves. Amniotic fluid is slightly thicker and more opaque than actual water and has a mildly pungent scent similar to semen. Amniotic fluid is NOT water as in H2O. So saying that a person's "water" breaks does not refer to actual water.

Often, a woman whose water breaks initially believes she has urinated. When examined under a microscope, amniotic fluid has a feathering effect. If there is any doubt about whether amniotic fluid is present in the vagina, a caregiver can check a sample under a microscope to confirm or use a type of litmus strip called "nitrazine paper" that reacts to the high alkaline levels of amniotic fluid but not to the high acid levels of urine. The paper is very pH sensitive.

The most common reasons a woman thinks her membranes have ruptured when they have not is that she has had some unexpected urine leakage (very common with the bladder compression of late pregnancy) or she took a bath and had pockets of bath water trapped behind the uterine wall, blocked by the baby's head. These small pockets of water can remain inside her body until the woman later stands up and starts to walk or the baby shifts positions.

When the membranes rupture, it could be a gush if the membranes rupture at the cervical area or it could be a small stream if the rupture is against the uterine wall.

Labor contractions are caused by a release of the hormone oxytocin from the pituitary gland. Oxytocin is also released when woman breastfeeds or has an orgasm. Each time oxytocin is released, it causes uterine contractions. As a woman progresses through labor, a self-perpetuating cycle called a "positive feedback loop" is established to keep *true* labor moving.

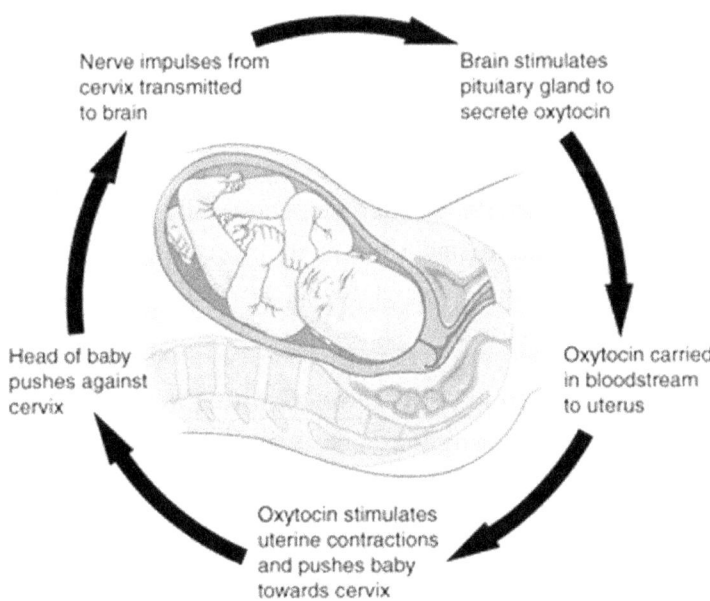

The Spiritual Aspect of Early Labor

When I was pregnant with my fifth child (fourth son), my water uncharacteristically broke as I was climbing into bed at midnight. It had been a lovely day, July 4th, and everyone except me was in bed for the night. I had no contractions to speak of yet, so I went into the kitchen and made myself a cup of sweet chamomile tea and since I had not eaten since early evening, I had some buttered toast and a spoonful of peanut butter. Sitting up in my bed, looking out my window at the night sky and drinking my tea, I felt a surge of empowerment and excitement. I knew something in that moment that no one else in the entire world knew: *my baby would be here by morning*. I was eight days early and with my other pregnancies, labor began days or weeks after my due date, so this was also unusual for me. My labors were only around two to four hours long once they got going, so I knew that by sun up, my baby would be here. I thought of all of those people sleeping, unaware of the miracle that was about to happen.

After an hour or so, I began to have contractions, so I phoned the midwife and let her know. Since I have my babies quickly, she said she would be right over. Then I phoned other people involved with the birth and settled in to wait for everyone to arrive.

It was a very potent, magical time. In that instance, I had the benefit of knowing that labor was starting because my membranes ruptured. There was no question that it was a membrane rupture. The darned thing just exploded and I was gushing like Old Faithful.

The moment when you realize that "this is not a drill" and false labor has given over to the real thing is a tremendously exciting and loaded moment. A place where television and movies get it right is that often, the pregnant woman is the one who is calm while everyone else around her is freaking out. Everyone involved should work to contain any sense of urgency and create a calm, peaceful environment around you. If contractions are uncomfortable, use your slow chest breathing (see Appendix 1 on Breathing Techniques) and active relaxation techniques to stay calm and loosey goosey.

Bond with your baby and send messages of safety, love, and welcome. If your partner is with you, spend time together as a couple or if you have other children, as a smaller family, enjoying those moments before the excitement and work of having a newborn sets in. Surround yourself with loving energy, smiles, and tranquility.

This is the easiest part of the laboring process, but it is also the longest. Second and third labors are usually half as long as first labors. Keep yourself open to whatever comes your way and fully trust that you have all of the resources to navigate the next few hours in health and strength.

Sleep absolutely as much as you can. A common concern of women in early labor is that they will wake up and find that they missed the birth. (That's adorable.) When your body needs your attention, it will let you know. You are about to enter the most profound athletic event you will ever experience and you need all of the rest you can get before it happens.

Of course, that can be challenging when you are filled with excitement over the impending birth. Practice your active relaxation and let it lead you into sleep if at all possible. Eat and drink lightly, but often, blessing every bite and drink you take toward the process of labor and delivery.

Know that you are participating in the sacred process that millions of your mothers and sisters before you have engaged. From life comes life and you are the conduit and creator of that life. Your DNA will now live on in this child, possibly for generations. Tune into the magnitude of what you are doing and know that you are fully capable of entering into that experience with strength and wisdom.

CHAPTER 6 – ACTIVE LABOR

During the active phase, the mother becomes more serious. There are still three to five minutes between contractions for her to communicate her needs, change positions, etc, but she is more internalized and less social than in preliminary phase.

Contractions are stronger when they occur and have greater duration, usually lasting sixty seconds or longer. Active labor normally kicks in when effacement completes. There is little question now that this is the real thing. In most cases, when active labor takes over, the laboring mom is uncomfortable enough that she seeks out her place of birth. If this place is home, she will usually want quiet, calm surroundings and to know that her midwife is on the way.

If the laboring mother has to transport to her place of birth, it is important to know that the motion of the vehicle while traveling will intensify the pain of contractions. The laboring woman should *not* attempt to drive herself to her place of birth. The driver should drive smoothly and carefully, remembering that the labor will progress whether the laboring mother is at her place of birth or in a car wrapped around a phone pole. Take corners slowly and carefully, jostling the mother no more than is necessary.

The goal is to get the mom to the place of birth after the long stretch of preliminary phase has ended and active labor is established, but before the extreme labor of the transition phase. Caregivers will have specific suggestions for when to come to the hospital/place of birth. Usually, it goes something like this: When **contractions are three to give minutes apart, lasting for at least sixty seconds *and have been in that established pattern for an hour or longer.*** Talk to your own prenatal health care provider to find out when they want you to contact them or come in when in labor. For a woman who has given birth before, the caregiver may want her to come to the hospital as soon as the contractions become regular, regardless of how far part they are coming.

A pregnant woman should always let her health care provider know:

*If the **membranes rupture** (to reduce the risk of infection since there is now access between the baby's immediate environment and the outside world).*

*If **bleeding** occurs that is bright red or is more than mild spotting.*

If she feels umbilical cord in the vaginal opening.

If the mom is able to walk during this phase of labor, it will generally go faster, regardless of her location.

There are two bags that are extremely important for the hospital stay. One is your labor bag or "goodie bag" and the other is your suitcase for after the baby is born. Both should be in the car with you when you go to your birthing place, but the suitcase stays in the car until you settle in your hospital room after the birth and the labor bag comes with you so you have your comfort tools available while you are in labor. You can find a full list of what to include in the Labor Bag and the Suitcase in Appendix 2.

Once the laboring woman reaches her place of birth and checks in, she will be taken to a labor area and made comfortable. I fully recommend a tour of your birthing place before you are in labor so you and your labor partner are familiar with the facility.

Some admission work may need to be performed, but most facilities used a "pre-admission" process that reduces paperwork upon actual admission significantly. A labor attendant will ask you questions about your labor so far. Here are some you will likely here:

Did your water break? When? How much was there? What did it look like?

How far apart are your contractions?

How long have your labor been going on?

When did you last eat?

When did you last go to the bathroom?

Have you seen any signs of your mucous plug?

An internal vaginal exam will be performed to determine your degree of progress in cervical effacement and dilation, as well as the station of the baby. If the baby's head is engaged, you may be allowed to walk around after admission, which can help stimulate labor. Walk and remain upright and out of the bed as much as possible. As labor progresses, if a woman lies down once, she will not likely get up again. It is easier to stay up and sit down in a chair, crouch by the bed, or hold onto your partner during a contraction than to lie in the bed. As soon as the laboring woman gets into bed, her labor contractions become less effective. This does not mean she should be tortured by keeping her out of bed if that is what she really wants to do. She has the final call.

If the option is available, I highly recommend laboring in a birthing tub. This is a tub that is sterilized and monitored by midwives or labor staff. I labored in a birthing tub for my sixth child and the pain reduction the warm water provided was amazing.

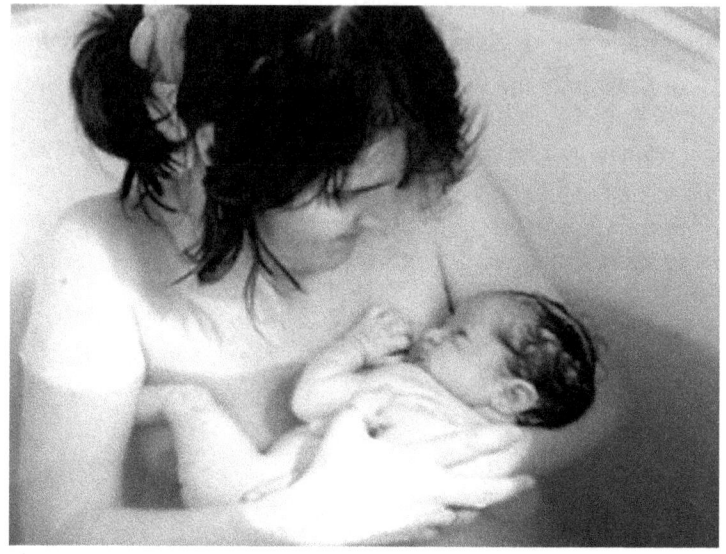

Both pushing and birth can occur in water with minimal risk to the mother or baby. Water births tend to be a gentler transition for the baby and a more comfortable delivery for the mother. Anyone interested in this option should research the practice and speak to their health care professional about it.

As labor becomes more intense, it is helpful to know that squatting often makes labor contractions more comfortable for women. Because of the softening of the fibrocartilage of the pelvis allows it to shift and move, squatting opens up the pelvic inlet and outlet a full twenty to twenty-five percent more than sitting or standing. This encourages the baby to descend lower and put more pressure on the dilating cervix, which causes labor to progress faster.

For most women, it is comfortable to squat while holding onto the bed or a support person. Since most people do not squat in their day-to-day activities as we did in the past, squatting for more than a few minutes can be uncomfortable. I recommend standing and leaning forward onto the bed, swaying your hips from side to side between contractions to help the baby move downward, and then holding onto the side of the bed and going into a squatting position for the duration of the contraction.

It can also be comfortable to kneel and sit with your knees apart and your butt between your heels. This accomplishes almost the same pelvic floor adjustment as actual squatting and can be comfortable if your legs do not lose circulation, remembering that blood flow centralizes into the abdomen during labor.

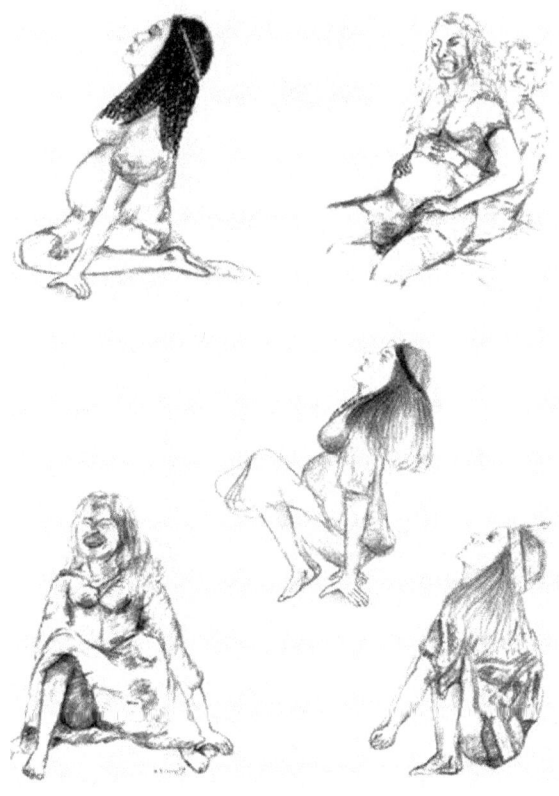

The previous chart shows some comfortable positions for labor that help the baby's head to make solid connection with the cervix and move downward effectively. Experimenting with different postures during labor helps to redistribute pressure of the baby's head to all areas of the cervix. This encourages even dilation and increases comfort.

A wonderful comfort tool is the birthing ball, which is actually a super strong exercise/balance ball.

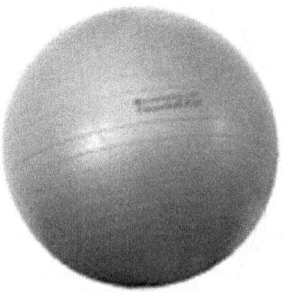

The laboring mother can kneel in front of the birthing ball and rest her elbows and a good bit of her body weight into the ball. She can also sit on the ball and emulate the position of squatting, while comfortably rocking back and forth to shift pressure from one side to the other.

Once the end of active phase approaches, the laboring mother focuses on herself and the labor process almost to the exclusion of anything else. There is usually very little conversation and she is not excited about the idea of changing positions.

When she begins to move into transition, the last phase of the first stage of labor, she will usually exhibit specific symptoms.

Dilation typically progresses from five to eight centimeters during this phase and the average length of active phase is three to five hours.

The Spiritual Aspect of Active Labor

When active labor progresses, you can truly feel the power of what you are doing and it is like riding a dragon. You feel fierce and unstoppable, but there is also the lingering fear that at any moment, this could all go off the rails and turn very, very bad. For most of active labor, you still feel in control, but the worry often begins to set in and it sounds something like this: *I am barely in control now. What happens if it gets worse? How can I take more?*

The most important thing you can do in active phase and transition is to stay strongly rooted in the power of *now*. Tap into your connection with the Divine and pull strength from the sky above you and the earth below you. With every breath, inhale peace and relaxation and exhale fear and tension. With every exhalation, become more and more relaxed.

Support people should time the contractions for you and let you know when a contraction has peaked and is on its way back down again. Laboring women often retain the memory of the strongest part of the contraction and do not realize when it is decreasing in strength.

Visualize your entire body opening up, releasing, and accommodating your baby's entry into the world. Breathe. Breathe. Breathe.

Focus on your focal point. As labor intensifies, it is very helpful to use your birthing partner's eyes as a focal point as they breathe with you. Doing so can help you to get lost in their focus and their love. It helps you to feel less alone to have a loved one right there with you, guiding your through the rough waters as the waves grow stronger.

Support people should pay particular attention to the shoulders and back in active labor as tension tends to collect there quickly. Minimize distractions and drama around her. Do not be afraid to say, "Not now, she is having a contraction." Be her advocate.

Another quick tension spot is the hands. Think of how we clench and unclench our fists when we are angry or in high emotion, how we drum our fingers when we are tense or anxious. To keep your hands relaxed during contractions, place your palms on your tummy and very lightly and gently make large circles around your belly. This technique is called effleurage (eff-loo-raj) and it calms the baby and keeps your hands relaxed. As your breathing speeds up into panting, keep your effleurage slow and in big circles, which gives you something else to focus on for pain relief.

A contraction now looks like this (see Appendix 1 for a full explanation of breathing techniques and practice them frequently with your support person before labor begins):

Contraction is coming.

Cleansing breath.

Relax your entire body.

Establish focal point as you exhale from the cleansing breath and remain locked onto the focal point visually until the contraction is over.

Use a patterned breathing technique of your choice throughout the contraction.

Keep your body completely relaxed throughout the contraction to allow your uterus to work without interference from surrounding muscle groups and to preserve energy.

Change to a higher level of breathing technique as the contraction builds if needed to maintain focus.

Your labor partner very gently checks for tension in your body and uses touch, voice, or both to encourage you to relax.

Shift back to a lower level of breathing if you can as the contraction releases.

Cleansing breath at the end.

Contraction is over.

Make necessary adjustments, wet your mouth, and change positions if needed before the next contraction comes.

For a full list of "labor tools," please see Appendix 3.

Between contractions, talk about what worked and what did not. Communicate to your support people what you need.

From active labor on, if the mother feels she needs to go to the bathroom, go with her in case she needs help. Sitting on the toilet can speed up labor because of the squatting position and our natural instinct to "release" when using the bathroom.

As you reach the end of this phase, you sometimes have mere seconds to tell your support people what you need to have happen. This can cause your words to become very clipped and direct. With my last baby, during a particularly intense set of contractions, I could only say, "STOP. MAKING. SOUNDS." The sound of my husband's voice as driving me mad and I wanted to choke him. He was only trying to help as we were taught, but it was distracting me from my focus.

CHAPTER 7 – COMMON MEDICAL PROCEDURES FOR LABOR

Although birth is a very normal process that occurred for thousands of years without medical intervention, there are still common practices a laboring mom can expect to encounter if she delivers in a hospital environment.

NPO – This is medical lingo for "nothing by mouth," short for "nil per os." Once a woman is admitted to the labor ward, she generally is not given anything to eat or drink until after the baby is born. This is done in case the woman needs general anesthesia for a cesarean. After the rush of delivery is over an hour or so after the baby's birth, the mom is typically *famished* and should be given food right away. During labor, most facilities allow the mother to chew on ice chips, popsicles, or suckers. Sometimes, juice or broth is allowed. This usually is not an issue unless labor goes on for a very long time. In that case, her reserves can definitely become depleted.

IV – Because the laboring woman is not eating or drinking, hospital still will usually insist on an IV line to keep her hydrated and to provide ready access to a vein if she needs medication.

Isolated to Bed – Some facilities do not allow the mother to walk during labor, especially if the amniotic membranes have ruptured citing a risk of infection.

Shaving – For many years, it was common practice to shave the mother's pubic hair. Multiple studies have shown that there is greater risk of infection from the shaving process than from the hair being present and most facilities no longer shave.

Enema – Some hospitals still require that the mother have an enema when she is admitted to clear the lower bowel. If the natural diarrhea has occurred, this may not be necessary. If the birthing staff can feel a good bit of stool in the bowel when they perform a vaginal exam, an enema can be helpful. A full bowel can cause pain in the lower back during labor and, let's face it, it is going to come out just before the baby. That kid's head is a snowplow.

Fetal Monitoring – All caregivers will want to monitor the baby's heartbeat during and between contractions, either intermittently or constantly. Some will simply check with the fetoscope or dopler, as illustrated previously in this book.

Some will want to use continuous monitoring, either external or internal. An external fetal monitor is attached to the mother's abdomen by velcro belts. One transducer rests on her lower abdomen to track the fetal heart tones and another, which has a pressure sensitive button on the bottom, goes on the top of her uterus to measure the strength of the contractions. This allows staff to see how the baby's heart rate changes during the stress of the contractions.

A record of the heart rate during and between contractions is created and a printed strip with this information will roll out. The monitor produces an audible sound of the baby's heartbeat and the volume of the heartbeat sound from the monitor can be turned down if it is distracting to the laboring mother. During the course of the labor, the baby will often move away from the transducer that picks up the heartbeat. This can be frightening to the mother if the baby's heartbeat is suddenly gone. Repositioning of the transducer will quickly find the heartbeat again.

If closer assessment is needed, the birthing staff may opt for internal monitoring. This is done by using a scalp clip electrode:

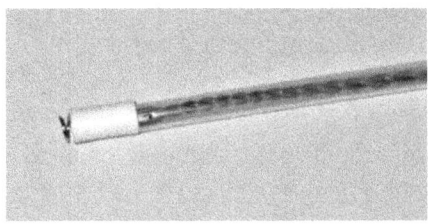

This electrode is attached to the baby's scalp by that spiral shaped pin screwing into the first few layers of skin on the baby's head. An internal pressure catheter may be used to monitor the contractions as well. It is a thin, plastic wand-looking device that slides into the uterus through the open cervix between the baby and the uterine wall. The membranes must be ruptured for these internal monitors to be used and the woman will be confined to the bed during their use.

Medications – Medications are usually a matter of preference for the laboring mother. There are different levels of medication available for her comfort. **Analgesics** are muscle relaxants that slow down the contracting of the uterus, resulting in less discomfort. These are usually administered through an IV. Obviously, if the strength of the contractions is diminished, the labor will be prolonged unless pain is causing the mother to tense enough to slow the labor herself through muscle interference with the contracting uterus.

Babies tend to go to sleep when an analgesic is administered and the heart rate drops considerably. Medication is given based on the weight of the mother, not the weight of the baby. This means the baby receives a dose significantly higher than it would receive for its own weight.

Demerol is one of the most commonly used analgesics in labor. Analgesics are rarely used after seven centimeters of dilation because after that time, birth is imminent and the baby needs time to metabolize the analgesic and pass it back through the placenta before birth.

Anesthetics are numbing agents that take away sensation. The most commonly used anesthetic for birth in the U.S. is the epidural:

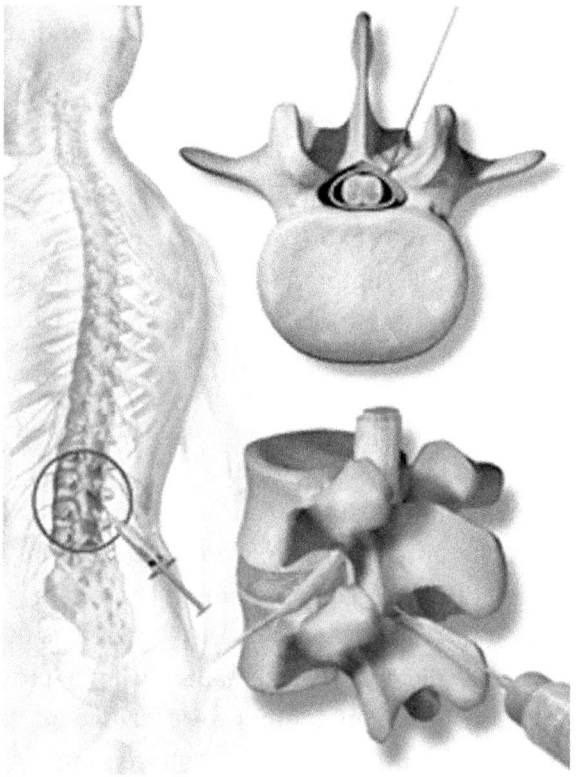

The laboring woman is given a local anesthetic and a catheter is inserted into the epidural space just outside of the spinal cord (lower back), through which an anesthetic is administered. This creates numbness from the breasts to the knees.

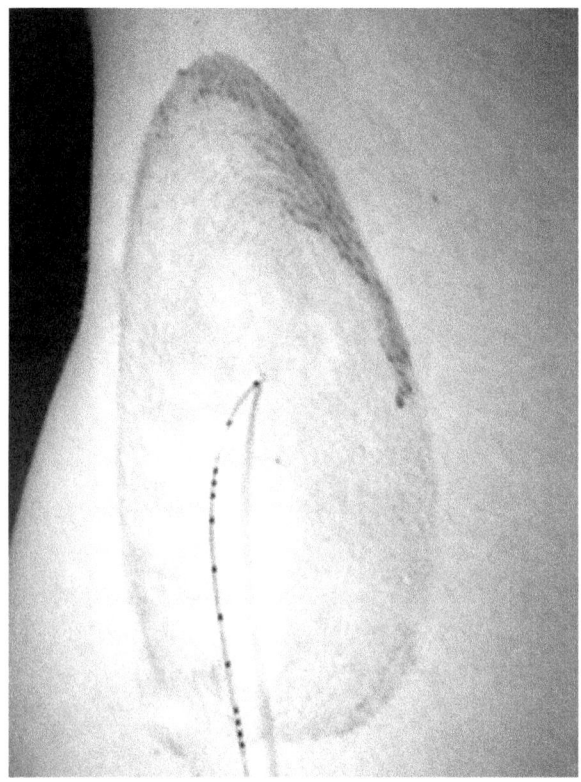

The catheter stays in place with a continual infusion for the duration of the labor until time to push. Laboring women often cannot effectively push if they are numb below the breasts, so epidural births often precipitate assisted births with forceps or a vacuum extractor.

When a spinal block is administered, the same process is used as with an epidural, but the catheter extends into the spinal fluid, which is more dangerous. Epidurals may also be used for a cesarean section to allow the mother to be awake for the surgery.

Another instance in which an anesthetic is used is for the **episiotomy**. An episiotomy is an incision made into the perineum to widen the birth canal and allow the baby to be born more quickly:

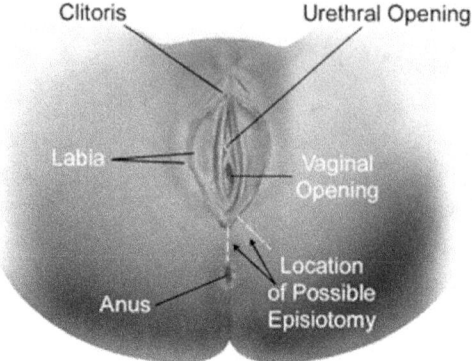

Clitoris Urethral Opening

Labia

Vaginal Opening

Location of Possible Episiotomy

Anus

Female Perineum

The episiotomy is done just prior to crowning and is stitched up after the placenta is delivered.

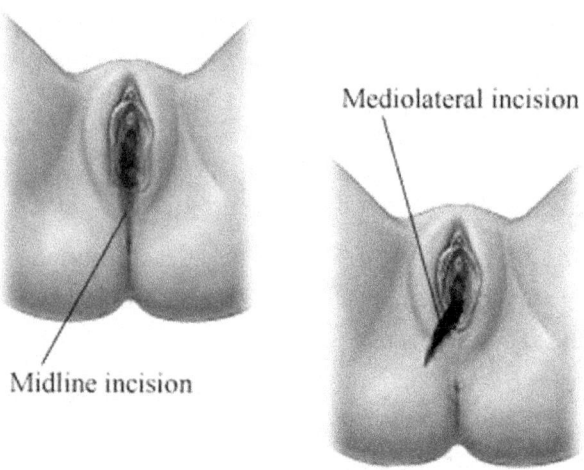

Mediolateral incision

Midline incision

Yes. Ow.

Most midwives and progressive caregivers no longer use an episiotomy unless it is necessary for the health of the mother or baby. The episiotomy is performed as the baby's head in crowning using a special type of scissors that is flat on one blade and sharp on the other.

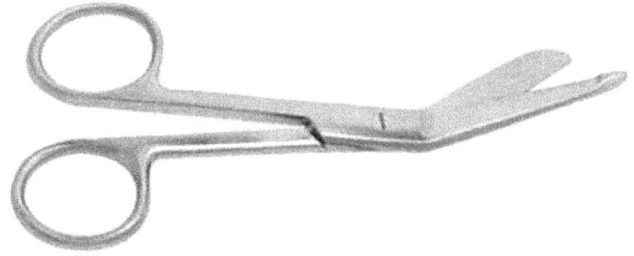

The baby's head cuts off a good bit of the blood flow into the perineum as it is crowning, so there is not a lot of blood at the time of the cut, but after the baby is born and the tissues begin to thicken again, the area must be stitched like any other surgical site. The pressure of the baby's head also seals off the nerve endings to the perineum, so the mother does not feel the cut happen. You can hear it, however, and it sounds a little like someone is cutting through corrugated cardboard.

Just prior to cutting, the attendant will inject an anesthetic (lidocaine or carbocaine, much like is used at the dentist's office) into the perineum to numb it. This is *not* numbing the area for the cut because the anesthetic will not take effect for several minutes and at this time, birth in imminent. It is for the stitching that will come later.

Having experienced my first birth with a mediolateral incision, my second birth with a midline incision, and my remaining four births with no episiotomy at all, I can vouch 100% for whole "no episiotomy unless absolutely necessary" route. If you are not in stirrups to deliver and If your birth attendant is performing perineal massage to help the perineum stretch around the baby's head, you most likely have a good chance of not needing an episiotomy. A birthing attendant can carefully observe and feel the perineum and tell if it is about to give way to a tear, then cut at the last minute if needed.

Some attendants automatically perform episiotomies as routine. This is an important point to discuss in your birth plan before you are in labor.

With my first birth, it was approximately three months before I could sit comfortably again. With my second birth, it was approximately two weeks. With the last four births, I could sit comfortably immediately after birth.

Ice packs to the episiotomy site immediately after birth help reduce swelling and pain.

The Spiritual Aspect of Medical Procedures For Labor

One might not believe there could be anything spiritual about routine medical procedures, but one of the greatest aspects of any spiritual connection is the balance between surrender and free will. That shift creates the tightrope we walk every day between being empowered and being a victim.

My opinions on the invasion of modern medicine into birth are likely clear from what I have written in the introduction of this book. Birth is a condition of wellness, not a condition of illness. Birth is an expression of perfect nature; not an emergency to manage.

When we go into the idea of birth shuddering and huddling together like frightened children over the ideas of what *might* happen, we become little more than campers with flashlights under our chins in the dark telling ghost stories. Are there complications with birth? Of course, there are. In fact, I have an entire chapter of this book devoted to what *could* go wrong, just so you are adequately educated about the possibilities.

Our medical system lives in terror of producing anything less than a perfect outcome and why? Because of the threat of malpractice suits that can end the career of a physician or bankrupt a hospital, depending on the severity. For that reason alone, any minor indication that something *might* be wrong causes the medical staff to fly into action. A laboring mother is very vulnerable to fear and worry, so placing her in an institution focused on crisis management can overwhelm her with concern. Fear breeds tension, which creates complications.

Consider this: A labor nurse looks at the results of the monitor strip and says, "The baby's heart rate is going down during your contractions." If the mother does not know that it is completely normal for the baby's heart tones to go down during a contraction, that can be terrifying to her.

This is why it is so essential that the pregnant woman trusts herself and her own body. Over centuries, we were trained out of believing that our bodies can birth naturally, normally, and safely. Society conditions us to believe that *something* will *always* go wrong and it is merely a matter of waiting for it and diligently sifting through every single reaction, every bit of evidence, waiting for that one tiny flaw that is going to cause the entire birth to go into the ditch.

From the moment she is pregnant, the expectant and laboring mother becomes an accident waiting to happen and the complications are not treated as the anomaly that they are by statistics, but as inevitability.

The fact that the vast majority of births are able to proceed normally and without incident or emergency is incidental. The fact that many of the aggressive medical procedures that do occur are actually caused by *other* medical procedures that were enacted *just in case* is also irrelevant to their thinking.

How is this spiritual?

Because if you look at the heart of this, it is all a head game. What is the most important factor in this entire process is *what the laboring woman believes to be true.*

A woman absolutely must be open minded to the idea that complications *could* occur and that if they do, we have the resources to manage them safely and effectively. Complications should *not*, however, be considered to be a foregone conclusion. The wise expectant mother educates herself about all aspects of childbirth and then proceeds into the process confident that she is fully capable of delivering a healthy, beautiful baby without incident.

Surrender and free will are complicated issues and are hard at work in the birthing process. One of the biggest differences between hospital births and home births is that a doctor or a hospital will tell you how things are routinely done in their facility and a midwife will ask you what you would like to have done for your birth.

Surrender is necessary because to gain the most from your birth experience, you must surrender yourself to the power of the labor and delivery. You must become one with it (please forgive the cheesy words, but there is really no better way to say it) and flow with it as though the birth process is carrying you along a swift river with many rapids. The river flows like this, easy and calm or rough and ragged, every single day. The river knows what it has to do and does it. Similarly, babies are born all the time, every minute of every day somewhere in the world. The birth process is very efficient and has been producing new people for as long as there have been people.

You however, have not been riding that river every day of your life and you have to find your way with it. You do so by relaxing and enjoying the ride, moving when the current moves and relaxing when it is calm.

Having worked on labor and delivery wards as a doula who is friends with every nurse also working there, I can tell you with some degree of authority that it is *much* easier for the staff when a laboring woman surrenders to the process of hospital policy and does not rock the boat. Routine deliveries are a blessing to the staff. The fact is, however, that surrender to hospital policy and offering yourself up meekly as a childbearing vessel for others to do with as they see fit is not always a wise way to birth.

Educate, educate, educate. Learn all you can about birth. Decide which routine procedures work for you and which ones do not. Establish your birth plan and then talk to your doctor or caregiver about it well in advance of the birth. Do not show up at the labor and delivery ward in active labor waving your birth plan without a doctor's signature on it and advanced planning. You can ask, of course, but making choices will in advance and then being open to change as it is necessary is always best. Your considerations might look something like this:

Barring extreme complications, I wish to deliver in a birthing room or in the labor room, not the delivery room.

I would like to forego the use of stirrups and to have the freedom to change positions during the pushing process.

I would like my birth attendant to perform perineal massage and only use an episiotomy if necessary.

I wish to be consulted before any medication is administered to me or to my baby.

I wish to wait for the IV to be inserted until I am no longer comfortable walking the halls of the hospital to stimulate labor.

I would like my birth partner to cut the baby's umbilical cord.

I would like to have intermittent fetal monitoring with a dopler instead of full-time monitoring unless there is reason for concern.

I wish to forego shaving or an enema upon admission.

I would like internal exams to be as infrequent as possible.

I would like to breastfeed immediately upon delivery.

These are just some ideas and each woman will have her own list of what is important to her. Some childbirth attendants will not budge on certain policies and it is up to the woman to determine, preferably before the thirty-sixth week of pregnancy, whether their birth attendant's policies are conducive to her own desires. There is no shame or harm in changing providers to find someone more in keeping with your personal wishes. After thirty-six weeks, the birth is coming up quickly and many professionals are uncomfortable taking on new clients that late in the pregnancy.

There are several reasons why pregnant women stay with health care professionals who do not support their own philosophies:

Their insurance only covers this provider.

Their mother or partner prefers this provider.

They are afraid their provider will be insulted or hurt if they are dropped.

They are afraid of change and of meeting a new provider.

They do not trust themselves to make good decisions about who should be their health care provider.

I am sure you can see how some of these reasons fall snugly into the "surrender yourself" mindset.

Free will is what you employ when you make your own choices in cooperation with your childbirth caregiver. A good caregiver will be open to your interests and will work hard to accommodate you. If you are delivering outside of your home, have your health care provider sign and stamp two copies of your birthing plan. One stays with you and one goes into your prenatal records. This tells the hospital staff that the caregiver is aware of and agrees to your requests.

Trusting yourself and the natural process of birth is a tremendously spiritual connection and frankly, it is does not come easily to most people. This is why the acts of meditation, thoughtfulness, affirmations, and education are so very important.

Remain completely grounded in confidence and assurance, but open to the wisdom of alternative intervention if it is necessary.

Be wise, be calm, be assertive when necessary, be confident in yourself.

CHAPTER 8 – TRANSITION

As the transition phase begins, several signs may manifest to alert the laboring woman and her support team that the first stage of labor is about to end. Support people should work very hard to tune into the needs of the laboring woman, to read her nonverbal communication, and to anticipate her needs without her having to voice them.

Hot sweats or cold chills - During transition, the body is working harder than it might ever work again to pull the last two centimeters, the "lip" of the cervix, past the baby's head. Because of this tremendous effort, the blood is really pumping. When the contraction ends, everything stops for a few seconds to a few minutes. It is common for the laboring mother to have hot flashes and sweat profusely during a contraction and then become very cold when the contraction ends and the blood flow suddenly slows down again. Support people should become very good with the cool cloths and blankets and never mix up the two. She will absolutely let you know what she needs and when she needs it.

Involuntary shaking/teeth chattering - The body produces a huge rush of adrenalin in anticipation of the pushing stage. Usually, this rush comes before it is time to push. Since the energy of the adrenalin has to go somewhere, it takes the form of profound shaking and chattering teeth. This unrelated to the mother's chills, but a warm blanket might help her psychologically since the mind tends to associate shaking with being cold. This shaking will often continue after the birth in order to discharge residual adrenalin.

Nausea and vomiting - This is common because of the near complete shutdown of the digestive system that occurs to accommodate the tremendous energy needed for labor.

Exhaustion – For obvious reasons. Women also become extremely groggy from a rush of endorphins and may doze between contractions. Be sure and wake her a few seconds before the next contraction begins to allow her a moment to prepare for it. Unlike a typical sleep cycle, she may dream a little as she goes into these weird mini-sleeps between contractions. Support people should not be surprised if she says odd things during transition that may come from dream fragments.

Vocalizing - Women will often begin to make very guttural, primal noises in labor. At this point in the labor process, women are extremely internalized and self-preserving. They are very direct about their needs and this can sometimes be unkind, even for women who are not typically so commanding. It is essential that the support team of the laboring woman not take personally her abrupt commands and barking orders. All attention of everyone in the room should be toward her total comfort, exclusive of her demeanor as she does this incredible work.

Cervical bleeding - From capillary rupture in the cervix and it pulls back. This will take the form of mild spotting.

Membranes rupture if they have not done so before.

Confusion, disorientation and an other-worldly, disconnected feeling from the surging hormones.

Feelings of doom or fear because their mind registers, "If this gets any worse, I can't take it." Continue to assure them that they are almost there, almost done, and that this is the most intense labor will get. Some women become very morbid during transition, convinced that they or their baby will die. Continue to reassure her that all is well, that she is doing great, and most importantly, "Almost there..."

The sensation of needing to bear down or have a bowel movement - This is from pressure of the baby moving into the birth canal. Although the function is different, it is much like having a severe urgency to have a bowel movement and having to fight it. The mother should not push until she is told her cervix is completely dilated. To avoid pushing, she should blow through her pursed lips. Pushing before complete dilation (except under the advice of her birth attendant) can cause bruising or tearing of the now ultra-thin cervix. This urge to push may exhibit involuntarily with the woman not realizing that she is doing it, so watch for grunting or bearing down that she does not realize she is doing. The compulsion is extremely overwhelming.

Health care professionals will usually *not* use medications during this phase of labor because birth is imminent and there is no guarantee that the baby would have time to metabolize the drugs and pass them back to the mother before birth. Babies born under the influence of a mom-sized dose of medication are very lethargic and slow to respond, which is a health risk for the newborn. The ideal time for administering medication is between five and eight centimeters dilation during the active labor phase. Ironically, transition is the time when if you were to take medications, you need them most.

Dilation during transition is from eight to ten centimeters. This phase usually lasts from a few contractions up to two hours or so. It is the shortest, but most intense phase of labor.

The Spiritual Aspect of Transition

There is likely no time that a laboring woman will be so far between the worlds without the use of drugs as she is in transition. Between the endorphins and adrenalin that course through you and the haze of pain, pressure, and power that you embrace, there is little time for anything from the outside world to penetrate your awareness. Every fiber of your attention turns toward breathing, focus, relaxation, and release. Sometimes, you will stop hearing people's voices.

Specific sounds might become very annoying to you.

You may find your skin becomes extremely sensitive to touch and you cannot stand for your partner to touch you or place cool cloths on you anymore. Some women tear their clothes off because the feel of the fabric is distracting to them. It is as though their wild woman calls and they answer.

A very primitive feeling comes over a woman while she is in transition. She is fully engaged in the process and nothing else exists for her. She is creating. She is raging. She is the Morrigan. She is Kali Ma. She is Hecate at the gates of Hell. She is every fearsome Goddess to ever cross the minds of humans.

Some women do not have pain with their childbirth, only discomfort. Most do find the experience to be painful and it takes all of that woman's focus to remain relaxed in her body so that her uterus can do its job unhampered.

There is no time for politeness, for social masks, or for pretending. For this reason, it is essential that when you plan your birthing support team, you only allow people in the room with whom you have a good relationship. Only include people with whom you share a bond of love and safety or when you begin to have those hormones coursing through you, *shit's gonna get real*. I have seen old arguments long resolved resurface, old hurts coming into strong focus, and painful betrayals revisited as all of those brain chemicals kick up dust from hidden trunks and cubbies in your head.

One of my mentors once said that no matter what, a woman "speaks her truths" when she is having PMS, going through menopause, or giving birth. At other times, we can force ourselves to push down our feelings and our hurts for the sake of social decorum. During those three times of life, there is no holding us back. The moon blossoms to fullness and floods every dark corner with light and revelation.

Standing in your own sacred truths is also a very holy moment, even in the midst of pain and incredible hard work. You are purely yourself in this time and no one can take that from you.

Your birth partner should be your total advocate at this time, so do NOT choose someone who is shy and cannot maintain assertiveness in a high tension situation. Your birth advocate should be able to say things like, "She needs some time without a crowd right now" or "Please wait a moment before talking to her. She's having a contraction."

Usually, labor staff will wait until you are not contracting to do a pelvic exam, however, there is sometimes a benefit to examining a woman during a contraction to see how far back the cervix pulls under the force of a contraction rather than when it is at rest.

During this incredibly powerful time, go with your own instincts and work with your support person to maintain control and pain relief during contractions whenever possible.

CHAPTER 9 – STAGE 2, PUSHING AND BIRTH

Once a labor attendant examines the mom and determines that the cervix is fully open (ten centimeters, about the size of a baseball), the mother may begin to push, and Stage 2 of the labor process begins.

Once pushing begins, the fogginess of transition lifts and the mother becomes awake, aware, and intent on her job of pushing. She is extremely focused and on task. While pushing, the laboring mother has a considerable reduction in the pain from her contractions. When she is not pushing, she will have a transition-quality contraction. The contracting uterus is no longer dilating the cervix, but is now working to push the baby out, much like pushing the bottom and sides of a toothpaste tube causes toothpaste to come out the end. The uterus exerts pressure from the top and sides onto the baby to shove it out of the cervix.

It is essential that the mother direct her energy downward for effective pushing rather than arching the back so that her energy goes up and out from her. Her body should be curved into a C shape for optimum pressure on the fundus.

There are several effective pushing positions:

Semi-reclined, leaning against a partner.

Standing and squatting with a support person on each side.

Squatting beside a bed.

Hands and knees.

On a labor bed, pulling down on a "birthing bar," which is a bar extending over the bed specifically designed for the mother to grasp onto while pushing.

If the baby's heart tones are not favorable, the mother may be asked to lie on her left side to push, which is more difficult, but gets more oxygen to the baby.

The classic pushing position of pulling back on the knees while semi-reclined is considered by most to be not only the least effective position, but also the least comfortable for the mom. Because of the angle at which the baby emerges, the classic position for pushing has the mother pushing the baby *uphill* after the head passes under the pubic bone. Also, the relaxin has softened the fibrocartilage in the pelvis to allow it to shift and move to accommodate the downward progress of the baby during pushing. When the woman is squatting or on all fours to push, the pelvis can move freely. When she is on her back or even semi-reclined, her weight rests on the sacrum, which is then unable to move to shift with the baby's descent.

Sitting in a more upright position helps, but is still not optimal. Unfortunately, this is the position most hospitals use for birth. It is, however, an important improvement over the previous decades of birth in the United States when women were strapped down flat on their backs with the legs in stirrups and told to push.

Fortunately, most birthing facilities no longer require laboring moms to lie on their backs when pushing. The delivery room is now mostly used if extreme labor complications develop.

A typical hospital delivery room is shown below:

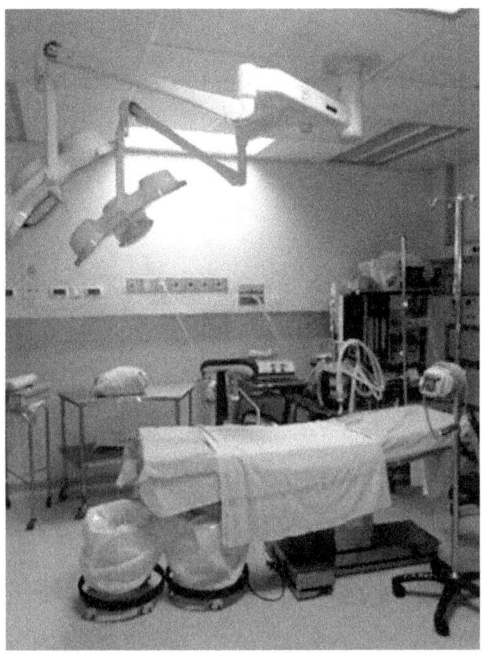

Some hospitals use birthing chairs or birthing beds. This is a birthing stool from long ago:

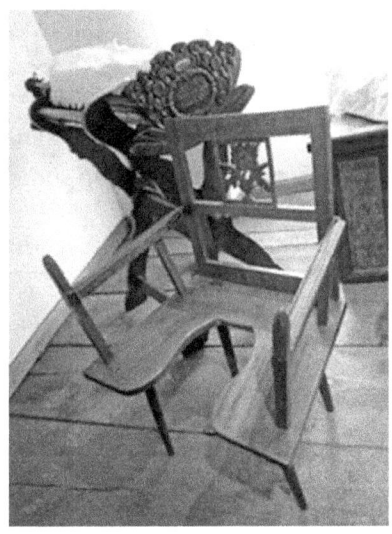

As you can see, it would be quite effective at supporting the mother in an upright position while allowing access for a birth attendant to catch the baby. ...and this is an ultra swanky, yes-these-really-exist, super-modern birthing chair:

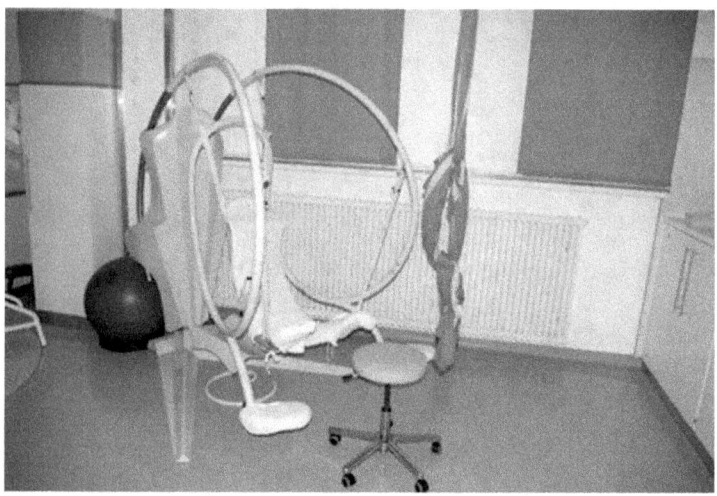

Notice that this birthing chair is actually a swing with foot supports for the laboring mom to use for counter pressure. What looks like a rag or bed sheet hanging from the ceiling is a strong support cloth for the mother to pull against to push while standing. (I would completely give birth in this place)

If labor is progressing normally and there are no signs of distress in the baby or mother, most birthing facilities will allow the mother to push in any position she chooses.

When a woman begins pushing, her caregiver starts a technique called "**perineal massage**." The perineum is the area between the vagina and the anus. Two fingers from each hand are inserted into the vagina and the lower posterior vaginal wall is massaged to help it stretch. A lubricant such as KY Jelly may be used to assist the massage. In home births, extra virgin olive oil is sometimes used. Perineal massage helps the vaginal tissues stretch around the baby's descending head.

During the second stage, the baby moves downward during the contraction while the mother is pushing. When the contraction ends and the mother stops pushing, the baby slips back slightly. The progression is akin to "three steps down, two steps back."

Toward the end of the first stage of labor, the baby turns so that the face is against the mother's sacrum.

As the baby descends, the usual position is face down (if the mother is on her back).

During contractions all through labor, the baby's heart rate (called **FHT** for "**fetal heart tones**") will slow down, called **"decelerations" or "decels,"** then bounce back after the contraction. This is particularly true during the second stage. Birth staff will keep close tabs on the FHT during and after contractions to make certain the baby is tolerating labor well.

Pushing can take anywhere from one or two pushes to three or four hours, depending on the circumstances. Women who have birthed before tend to have shorter pushing times. After having several children, the fundus becomes less muscular and may eventually revert to longer pushing times again.

Once the baby's head has slipped under the pubic bone, it will no longer slide back between contractions. The part of the baby's head that a crown would sit on is circled by the pubic archway. This point is called **"crowning."**

The anus will often become distended at this time. It is not unusual for a woman to have a bowel movement as she is pushing as the baby's head shoves everything out that is in front of it. The baby never comes into contact with the poop because of the thin rectovaginal wall that separates the rectum from the vagina.

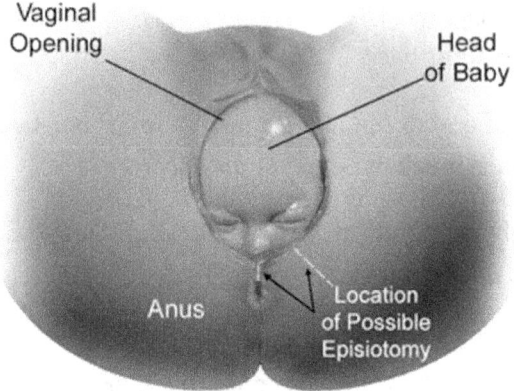

A very glistening image of crowning without the usual distractions of poop, a bit of blood, and pubic hair. This is how it looks on the outside.

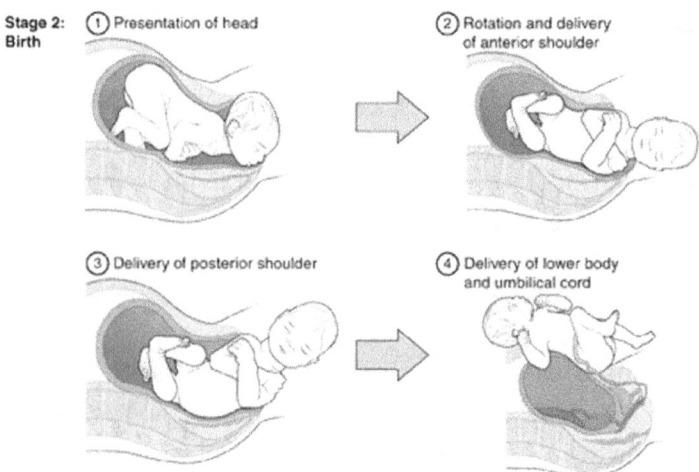

At the moment of crowning or just before, the woman will usually experience an intense, but brief, burning/stinging sensation called a "**ring of fire**." This tremendous sensation occurs when nerve endings of the vaginal opening react intensely just before going numb from the pressure of the baby's head. This renders the entire vaginal opening numb for the remainder of the birth process. Most women will gasp and stop pushing when the feel the ring of fire, which allows the head to birth gently instead of forcefully.

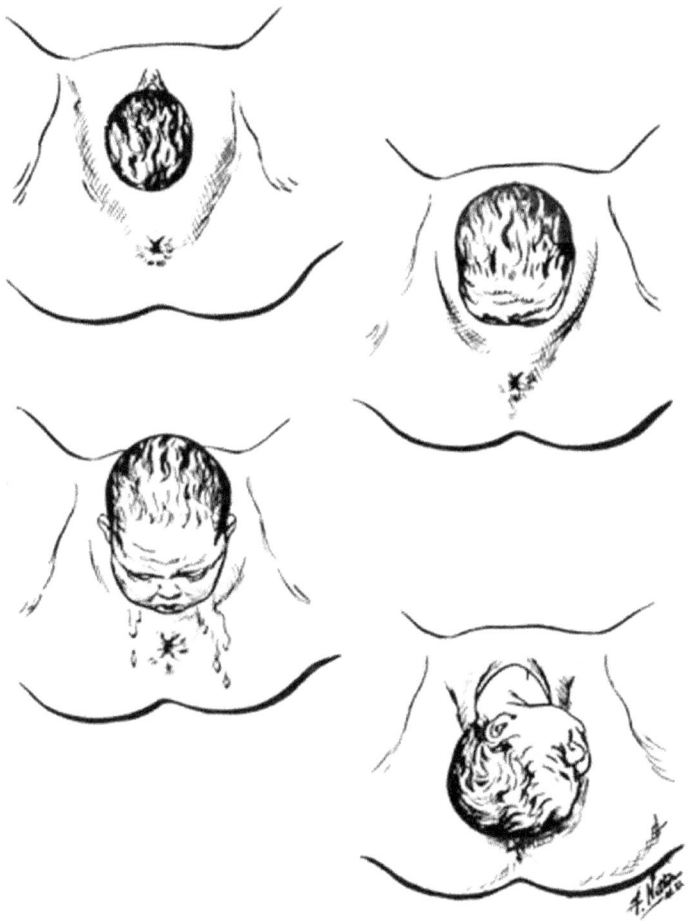

What birth looks like from the outside.

On the push after crowning, the head will be born and arch upward as the neck passes under the pubic archway. The baby's eyes may be open or closed.

On the next push, the baby's body will rotate inside, causing the head to turn on the outside. It will look as though the caregiver is turning the baby's head when they are actually supporting the head as it turns naturally.

On the next push, the top shoulder emerges and the baby will swoosh out of the body. The mother immediate feels a huge rush of relief and near absence of pain. Excess adrenaline will often cause the mother to shake dramatically and have chattering teeth at this time and possibly for up to an hour or so after the birth.

Despite what you may have seen in movies or on television, most babies are not very messy when they are born unless they are born early or late. Term babies are usually quite clean at birth and very warm. Their bodies "pink up" very quickly, starting at their chest with the newly oxygenated blood moving the "pink" from their chests to their extremities.

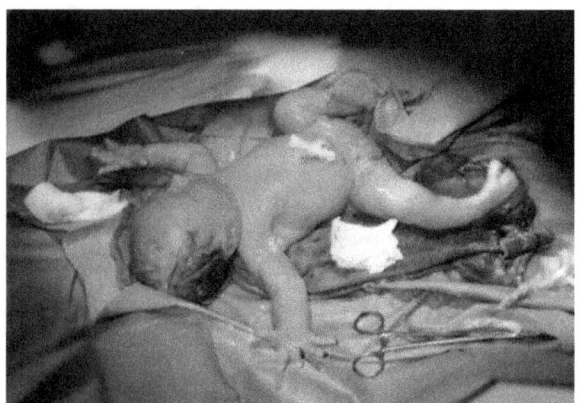

Average wet, messy baby before clean up, nice and pink

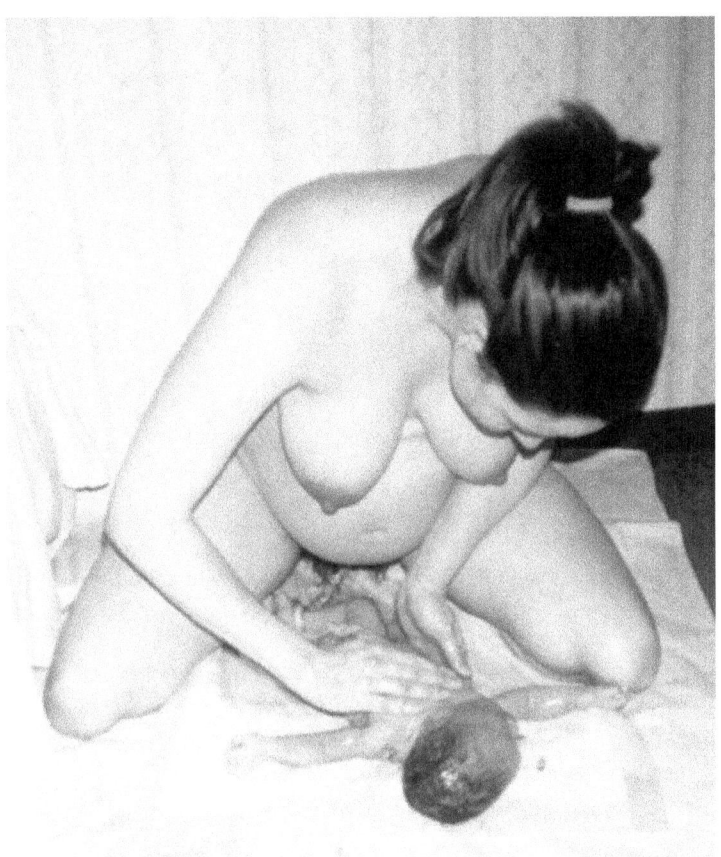

A mother stimulates her baby to help it pink up immediately after birth

Newborn faces are smushed from the passage through the birth canal. Premature babies usually have a shortening like substance on them called 'vernix caseosa.' Vernix keeps the baby's skin from deteriorating in the amniotic fluid. As the baby approaches the due date, the vernix starts to go away. If the baby is overdue, the vernix has been gone for a while, so the skin tends to be very peely. Vernix is a blood magnet and picks up lots of capillary blood during the birth passage. Birth itself is not usually very bloody until the placenta detaches and is born in Stage 3.

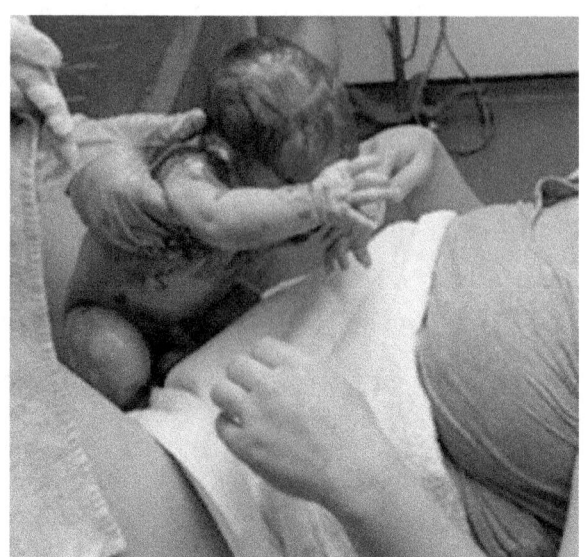

*This baby is bloodier than usual and the blood is bright red,
meaning Mama had a good-sized episiotomy*

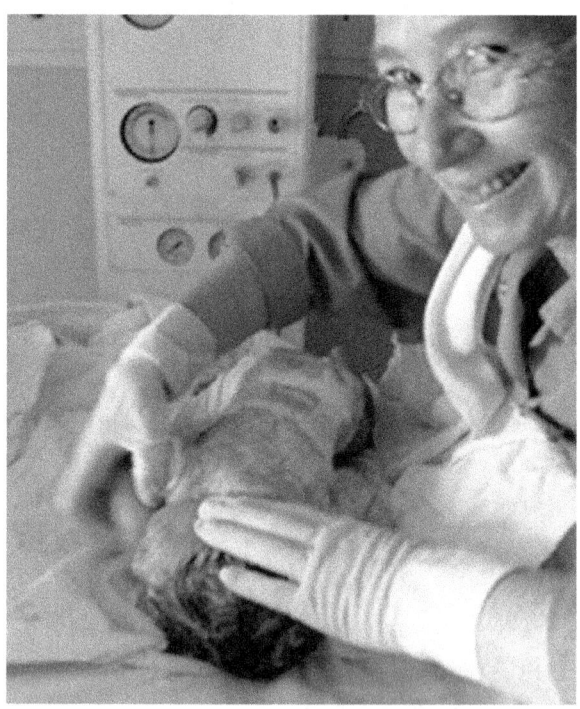

A premie with tons of vernix

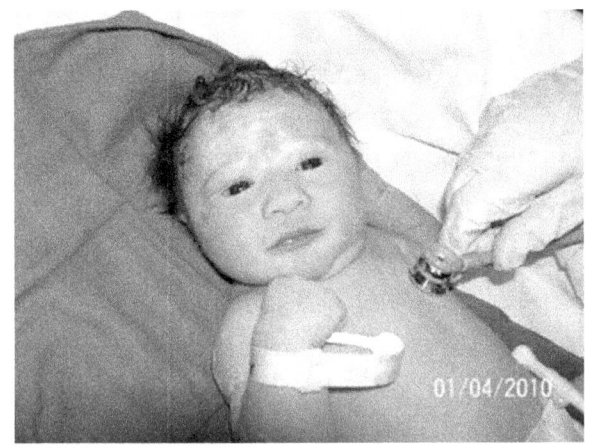

A newborn with vernix on his forehead and upper shoulder

Newborn babies may or may not cry when born. Whether they cry depends on how much trauma they endured with birth and their overall nature. Some kids are just screamers. The baby's head will likely be **"molded,"** which means pushed into odd shapes by the birth canal. The baby's **fontanelle**, also called a "soft spot" helps reduce pressure and allows the skull bones to overlap as it moves through the birth canal.

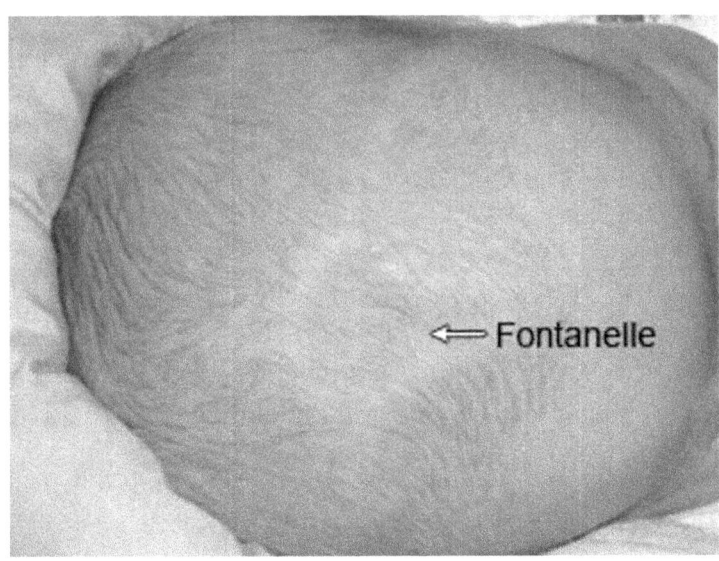

There are actually two fontanelles on the baby's head with a suture line that runs between them. This will close by the time the baby is approximately two-years-old. In the representation above, the face is to the right. The second fontantelle is in the top back of the head.

When a baby is born, they often do not immediately take a breath. They will continue to receive oxygen from the umbilical cord for as long as the placenta remains attached. If the baby does not take a breath within the first three to four minutes of life, the birthing staff will administer gentle encouragement such as stroking the cheek or bottoms of the feet, talking to the baby, rubbing the baby's head, etc. If the baby's oxygen has been compromised during the pushing stage, it might take the baby a few minutes to respond. Mucus will be suctioned from the baby's mouth, nose, and throat. This sometimes occurs as soon as the head is born in anticipation of the first breath.

Newborns normally want attention from the mother immediately and respond well to her caresses and to nursing. Breastfeeding immediately after birth assists with a cleaner placental separation. The hormone oxytocin releases when breastfeeding occurs and this causes the uterus to contract, which helps the placenta release from the uterine wall.

In a hospital birth, it is often an automatic procedure to put a shot of "pitocin," (synthetic oxytocin) into the mother's IV immediately after birth to help her uterus contract. If you do not want this, be sure and a statement in your birth plan that it should not be administered automatically, only "if needed."

The umbilical cord is naturally covered with a substance called **Wharton's jelly** that causes it to begin contracting down onto itself, cutting off the blood flow between the baby and the placenta.

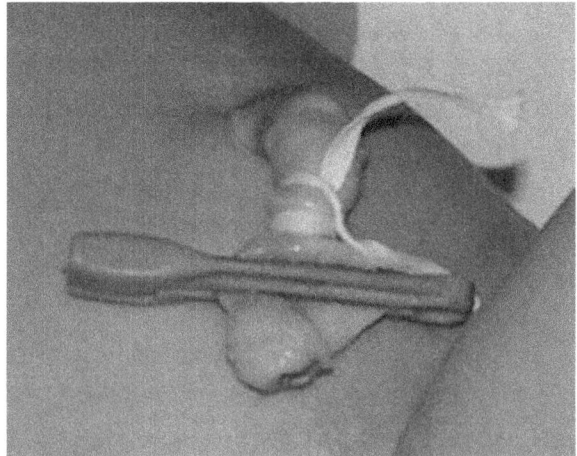

The umbilical cord will be clamped in two places, usually once it has stopped pulsing with blood. The cord is cut between the two clamps so that the mother does not bleed from the maternal end and the baby does not bleed from the navel.

The umbilical cord remains attached to the baby's navel for several days until it dries up and falls off.

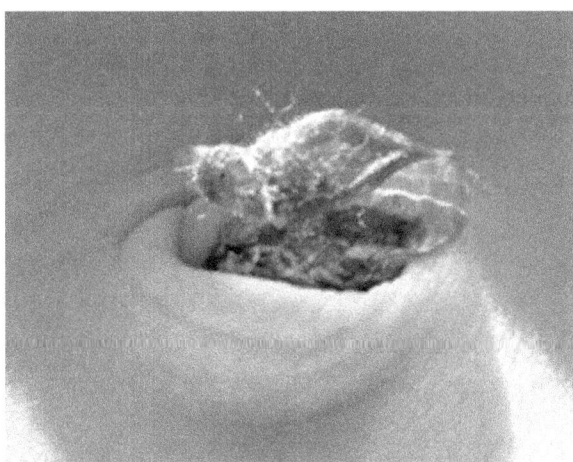

Under the cord stump is what will become the baby's belly button. Whether the baby has an "innie" or an "outie" is determined by genetics, not by the way the cord is cut.

For many years, there was a trend toward "milking" the blood that remains in the cord into the baby. Unfortunately, this practice caused a higher instance of jaundice in newborns because of the excess red blood cells the practice created. Unless there is a medical issue in which the baby must be quickly treated, the recommendation is to allow the cord to condense and stop pulsing, then clamp and cut the cord provided the baby is breathing well. Most umbilical cords are long enough that a mother can effectively nurse her baby without creating tension on the cord if the placenta is still attached.

One of the greatest fears in childbirth is that there will be cord around the baby's neck as it is being born. Media and books portrayed this as a major incident of concern when in reality, it is so commonplace for the cord to wrap around the baby's neck that most birth attendants do not even mention it. The cord is rarely tight and general practice is to have the mother blow instead of pushing through a contraction or two and gently ease the slippery cord over the baby's head until it is no longer around the neck. I have personally watched birth attendants move four or five loops of cord from around a baby's neck without incident. The greatest concern comes with very, very long cords that wrap around the baby's body and will not allow it to descend without a reduction of oxygen. This is indicated by reduced FHT and lack of progress in pushing and would usually require a cesarean section. Sometimes, a baby is born with a knot in the cord, such as my sixth child.

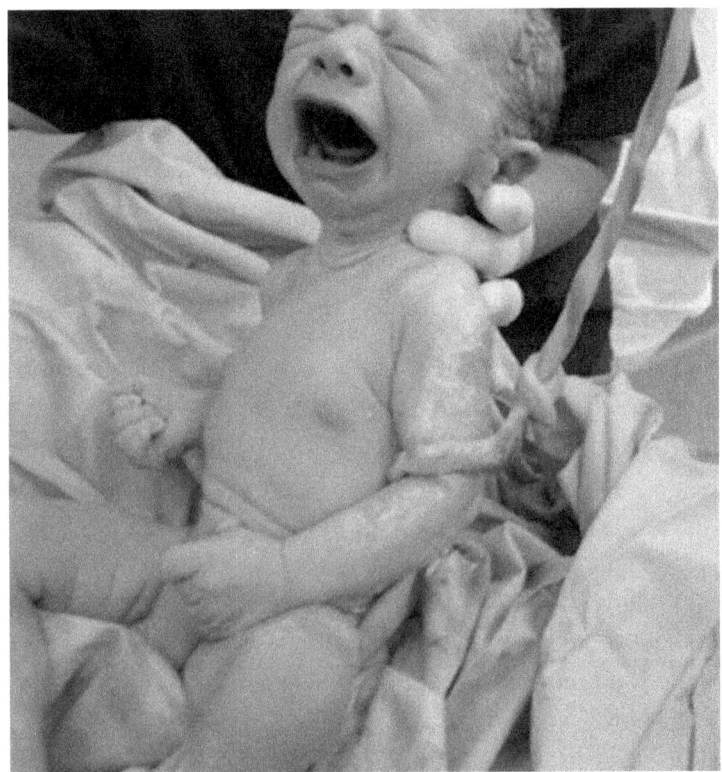

Baby with a true knot in the cord who seems PISSED about it

The Spiritual Aspect of Stage 2

Pushing can be a crazy exhausting task, but unlike Stage 1 of labor where we must remain passive and calm, surrendering to the process of labor and letting it flow through us and around us, when the time comes to push, we are suddenly very engaged and active. We are able to do exactly what our bodies tell us to do. For most women, there is a tremendous urge to push that manifests toward the end of transition and giving into it feels *wonderfully gratifying* and creates a near complete relief from pain.

The sensations one feels pushing a baby down and out are incredible. A big rush of energy comes in and you feel as though you could move mountains. There is a strong feeling of "waking up" from the dim, out-of-touch disconnection of transition.

This is a time of tremendous power and if you focus that power efficiently, you can crank this baby out in no time. Try not to be overwhelmed by how different this part of childbirth feels from the first stage. Just go with it and harness that power!

As your contraction begins, take two deep, quick breaths in and out of your mouth to get a boost of oxygen to your uterus and your baby as you begin to push. Remember that when you hold your breath, the baby's oxygen supply cuts off. Take another fast, deep breath and PUSH.

Remember to focus your power downward. It is normal to make primal, grunting sounds while pushing, but try to avoid loud, intense vocalizing, which uses energy you need for pushing.

Regardless of your position, turn your body inward and force your diaphragm down against your uterus, then push as your body tells you to push.

Try this experiment now: Take a deep breath and let it out quickly, saying the word "Pahhh" while you tighten your abdominal muscles. Feel how everything pushes down on your uterus? *That* is what you want to do when you are pushing.

As much as baby pushing is compared to having a bowel movement, it really is only that the sensation is similar. The action is very different. Push *into your vagina*, not your rectum. Visualize your body opening and releasing the baby, carrying it forward into the world on waves of maternal power.

For some women, pushing feels really great and by "great," I mean *really* great. Occasionally, woman will orgasm as the baby pushes past the G-spot (Grafenberg spot – a bundle of nerve endings in the inner, upper vagina – look it up, seriously). Since childbirth is actually a part of sexuality, you should never feel ashamed or embarrassed by the natural sensations you feel as it occurs.

We should all be so lucky. (sigh)

CHAPTER 10 – STAGE 3, BIRTH OF THE PLACENTA, PLUS SOME STAGE 4, FOUR HOURS RECOVERY TIME

After the baby is born, attention shifts to the placenta or "afterbirth." It will detach from the wall of the uterus between one and thirty minutes after the baby is born. The mother will likely feel some contractions as it works its way loose, although they are generally not uncomfortable.

Some hospitals will give the mother a shot, usually into an IV, of a drug called "Pitocin" as soon as the baby is born to cause the uterus to contract more aggressively and release the placenta. Breastfeeding has a similar effect since Pitocin is a synthetic form of oxytocin, the hormone that causes the uterus to contract in labor, while breastfeeding, and when the woman is sexually aroused. For bonding and contracting purposes, it is recommended that the mother breastfeed as soon after birth as possible, e*ven if she does not intend to continue breastfeeding after she leaves the hospital.*

When the placenta separates, there will be a gush of dark blood from the vagina. The separation of the placenta leaves a large, bleeding wound inside the uterus. It is essential that the now smaller uterus contracts down onto the placental wound to prevent hemorrhage in the mother.

Seriously, you and your support person should both prepare yourselves for the birth of the placenta because it is absolutely the craziest thing you will ever see. The side of the placenta that faced the baby is smooth, shiny, and purple with veins running through it. The side that was attached to the uterus looks a lot like ground beef, the expensive ground sirloin kind, not the cheap stuff.

Consider the fact that you have pushed an internal organ out of your body and trust me, the placenta does not disappoint. The umbilical cord still connects to roughly the middle of the placenta and amniotic membranes extend out from all sides of the placenta, forming a kind of soft fishbowl with a hole that the baby emerged from to be born.

It looks like this:

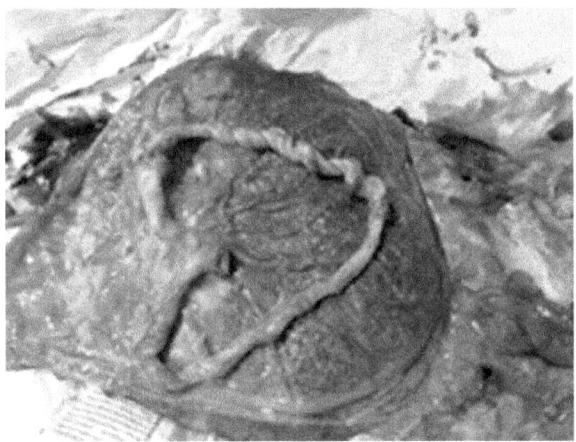

Veiny baby side

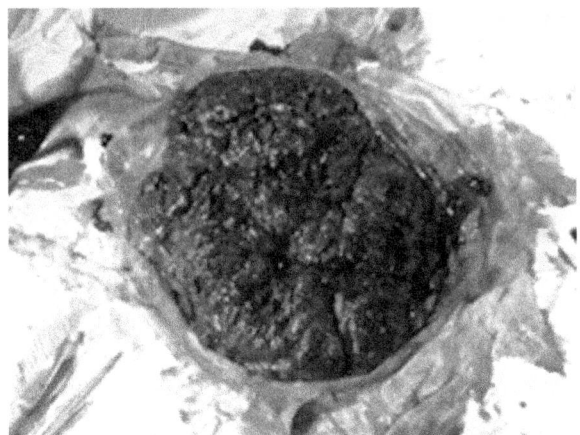

Beefy uterine side – the attendant will check the lobes to make sure the placenta is intact

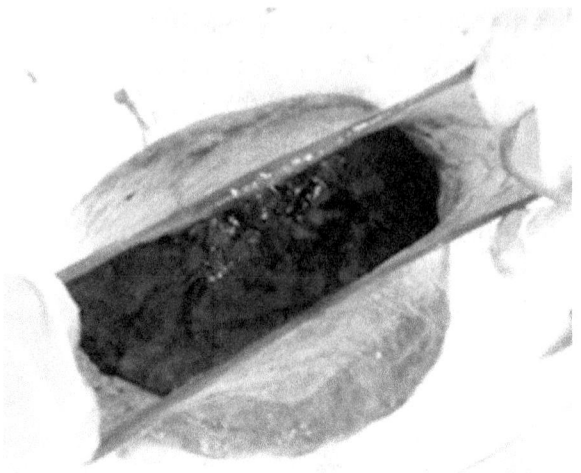

And here is the hole in the membranes where the baby came out.

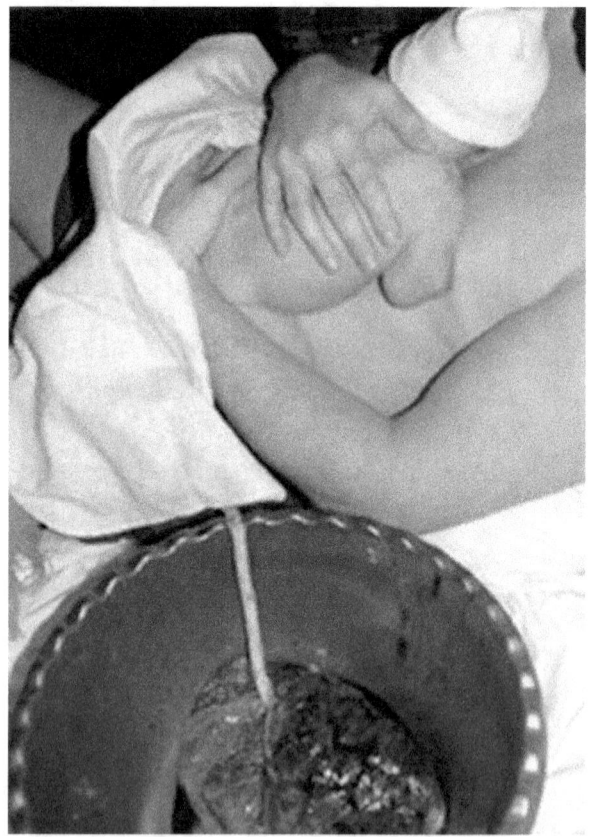

Baby with cord still attached, placenta to the side

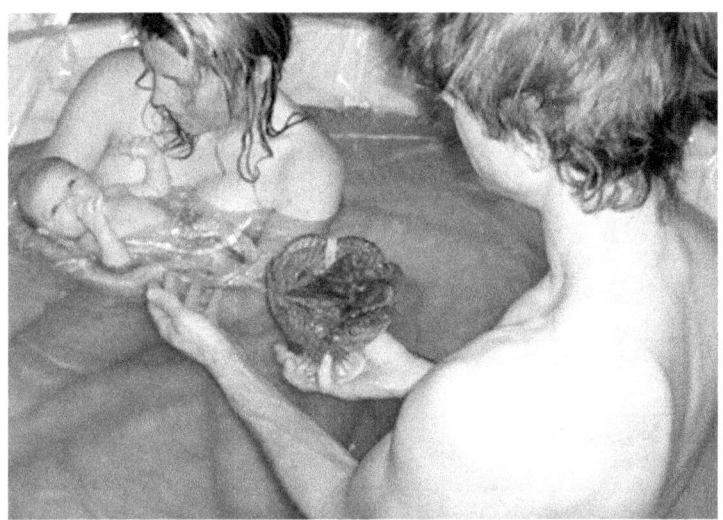

This baby born via water birth. You can clearly see the difference in the umbilical cord underwater (no air exposure, still blue) and attached to the placenta (white and deflated)

The birthing staff will massage the uterus from the outside, through the mother's abdomen, to encourage it to contract and will encourage the mother to do so herself. The uterus is very sensitive to touch and will contract when manually stimulated.

The placenta itself is caught in a specimen bowl and inspected carefully to check for any missing pieces that may still be inside the uterus. The placenta, membranes and umbilical cord will all be expelled with no part of the pregnancy left inside in the mother's body. The mother will continue to bleed on par with a very, very heavy period over the next three to four weeks. Some mothers, particularly those who have had children before, will have "afterpains" or cramping sensations for the first week or so postpartum, especially when they breastfeed. The shaking from transition will likely return once the baby is pushed out and because of the sudden slow down of blood flow in the body now that labor is over, the mother might feel cold.

At both one minute and five minutes after birth, the baby will be examined and given an **Apgar Score.** The Apgar Score is an immediate assessment of the baby's health. It was developed by a pediatrician, Virginia Apgar, and is used almost universally in the United States. The baby receives a score of 0, 1, or 2 points in the following categories:

SIGN	0	1	2	1 min	5 min
Heart Rate	Absent	Less Than 100	Over 100	2	2
Respiratory Effort	Absent	Slow, Irregular	Good Cry	1	2
Muscle Tone	Limp	Some Flexion	Active Motion	1	2
Reflex Irritability	No Response	Grimace	Cry	1	2
Color	Pale	Body Pink, Extr. Blue	All Pink	1	2
TOTAL SCORE				6	10

A baby with an Apgar of 8-10 is doing well and considered very healthy. A score of 4-7 is cause for concern and an Apgar of 3 and below is a baby in distress. Often, a baby with a lower score at one minute will have a healthier score at five minutes, as you can see above. An Apgar is recorded on the baby's records in the format of "4,8" with the first number representing the one minute score and the second number representing the five minute score.

In a hospital, staff will usually take the baby to an electric warming table or warmed bassinette for the newborn exam. Modern practice works to reunite the mother and baby for bonding as soon as possible and maximize the effects of the "quiet alert time" the baby exhibits within the first two hours of birth. Initial breastfeeding at this time is considerably helpful in imprinting the practice on the baby.

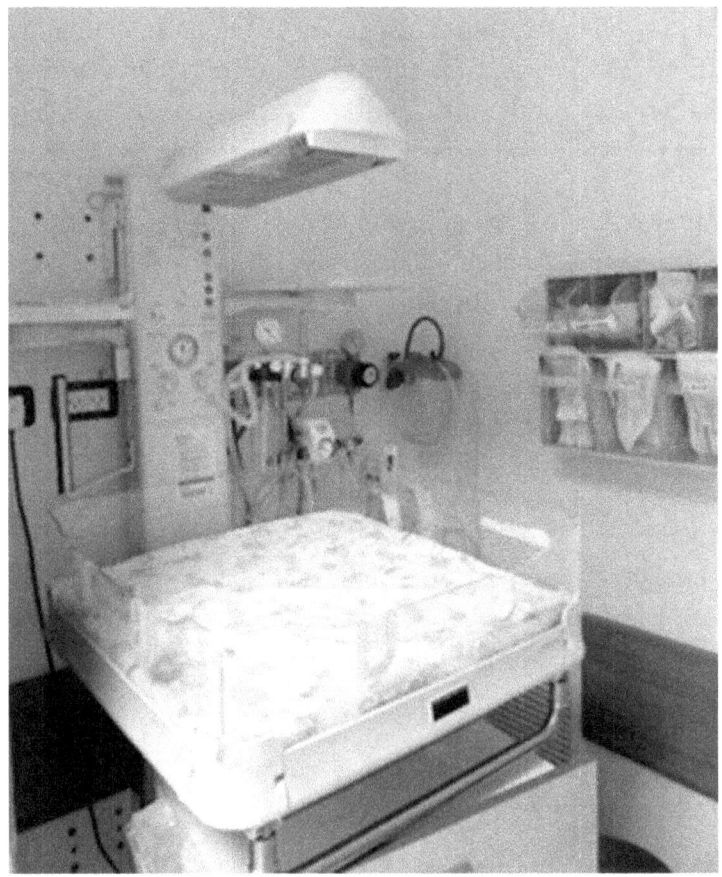

Baby Warmer

The birthing staff now has two patients to manage. Once the placenta is born and the mother's risk of hemorrhage is managed, the mother will be stitched if needed and cleaned up a bit. She will then have a sanitary napkin the size of a twin mattress placed between her legs and be wheeled either into a recovery room or taken to her postpartum room which she will occupy for the remainder of her stay. If the baby is healthy and stable, they may both room together, which is usually preferred. Health care staff will periodically check for vital signs and to make certain the uterus is well contracted onto the placental wound.

THIS is when the support person needs to make time to go to the car and *get that suitcase*. Mom is going to want a hairbrush, a toothbrush and toothpaste, a shower, possibly some makeup, and some excellent food *as soon as possible*.

Three hours before I went into labor with child number five, my future husband went back to his barracks and fell asleep around midnight with the phone in bed with him in case I called. He slept through the many phone calls and therefore, slept through the birth and woke up around 9:00 AM to learn that he had a son.

As I rested in my bedroom with my beautiful new little baby sleeping by my side, I looked up to see an arm sticking through my door waving a McDonald's bag, with sad puppy dog eyes behind it. Bring me hamburgers and I will forgive you anything and let me tell you, those were the best hamburgers I ever ate in my life.

As a hint, bringing back donuts, cookies, or other goodies for the staff goes a long way.

Staff will check your vitals and your uterus frequently over the next four hours. A lactation consultant may come in to make sure that breastfeeding is going well and to offer suggestions. Your IV will be removed shortly after birth if you have no further need of fluids or medications.

At some point, your baby will undergo a more thorough evaluation than the Apgar provides, including weighing, reflex testing, and feeling the hip joints and other body parts to make sure everything is where it is supposed to be. They will also be footprinted and your thumbprint will likely also be required.

Many hospitals automatically give the baby a shot of Vitamin K to promote clotting (you can refuse this, but be sure and tell them beforehand) and put an antibiotic in their eyes to prevent blindness from gonorrhea. Silver nitrate used to be used for this and it actually burned the baby's eyes to the point that they could not see and their eyes were red and puffy. Many thought this was from the birth, but babies who have Ilotycin cream instead do not have this. Interestingly, a baby's best eyesight focus is around 12-13", the distance between mom's crooked elbow and her eyes.

Circumcision is not as common for newborn boys now that it is known that the foreskin has a specific purpose, protecting the sensitive head of the penis from ammonia burn from urine, and that there is no longer a medical indication supporting the surgery.

Most mothers are able to check out of their place of birth within twenty-four to thirty-six hours of giving birth.

The Spiritual Aspect of Stages 3 and 4

This is an exuberant time of bonding and excitement as you finally get to see your new baby.

Some mothers and/or fathers like to "mark" the baby on the forehead with a thumbprint of birth blood as a blessing. Immediate nursing is very helpful at this time. Hold the baby close to your breast and tickle the corner of its mouth with your nipple. The baby will instinctively turn and root for the breast. When the baby's mouth opens, push as much of the nipple and areola into the mouth as you can.

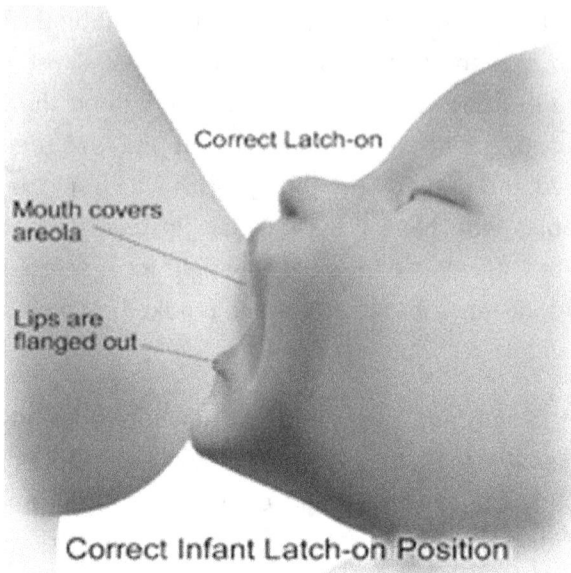

Correct Latch-on

Mouth covers
areola

Lips are
flanged out

Correct Infant Latch-on Position

You may be very surprised by the strength these little suckers have in their mouth and jaws. Once they latch on, you will know it! Nursing encourages good contractions of the uterus, which provides tight pressure on the placental wound site.

During the first two hours after birth, your baby is in what is called a "quiet alert" phase where it takes in all that it see in this new, alien environment. During this time, baby will seek out your eyes and your closeness for comfort. Your voice and the voice of those closest to your baby are very familiar, to talk to your baby and say welcoming, warm things.

Many people have asked me, "What do you do with the placenta when you have a home birth?" In a hospital birth, of course, the placenta is bio-waste and is disposed of in their special bio-waste bags. At home, however, there are a number of things you can do. Some people have a pre-dug hole in the yard and will put the placenta in the hole and plant a tree over it. The tree then becomes the baby's birth tree. Some midwives keep the occasional placenta, with permission from the parents, of course, to use for demonstration purposes in childbirth classes. A frozen placenta will keep for a very long time.

You may have heard of certain cultures eating the placenta. I can tell you that it is usually boiled, it is an offense to not partake, and it tastes a lot like tough liver.

Mostly, the placenta goes into a white trash bag and into the garbage, trusting that the trash man does not get overly curious.

The placenta is not the most attractive aspect of birth, but it is one of the most vital because it has effectively kept your beautiful baby fed and nourished for the past many months. I recommend checking it out because it is tremendously interesting. Men in particular seem drawn to them in that little boy "show me your scraped knee" way.

Over the next few days, you will likely be surprised by how good you feel. Most women do not realize how exhausted and uncomfortable they were during the last weeks of pregnancy until they have given birth. It can also be stunning after the discomfort of labor to have the pain suddenly stop. Be careful not to do too much too soon. Make sure you have people to help you in your home while you recover. Your focus should be solely on you, your baby, and a great deal of sleeping. You will have plenty of time to get other things done. For now, update your Facebook status and rest.

CHAPTER 11 – COMPLICATIONS OF CHILDBIRTH

As I have mentioned previously in this book, it is rare that hospitals or the medical profession acknowledge that childbirth is usually an uncomplicated and very natural process. Women have largely handed over the management of their pregnancy and birth to the medical profession, primarily men, who complicate a natural process to the point that it is now approached from a position of tremendous fear with the expectation that something will go wrong rather than honoring the overwhelming odds that no complications will occur.

Most medical procedures are initiated from a perspective of "but what if..?" rather than allowing nature to take its course and gently assisting the process if needed. Women are referred to as "patients" and placed in a hospital with those who are ill and dying rather than pregnancy being treating as a condition of health and vitality.

The movement of birth away from midwives and home care is what caused the epidemic of "childbed fever" that plagued the world for *two-hundred years* between the years 1600-1800. During this time, women gave birth in "lying in" hospitals tended by doctors who would return from dissecting cadavers to deliver babies with no form of antisepsis between the two procedures. Infections were rampant and maternal mortality skyrocketed.

Fortunately, the mindset of many childbirth institutions has become more accommodating of the natural processes and women often are able to have a satisfying birth in a hospital without excessive medical intervention.

In the United States, the maternal mortality rate for childbirth is 9-10 out of every 100,000. Worldwide, half a million women die in childbirth every year. In modernized countries, the infant mortality rate is approximately 1% of babies born between 28 weeks gestation and those who survived for up to 28 days old after birth.

As you can see, it is rare for a birth to reach a critical point of mortality for either mother or the baby. There are medical complications that do arise and both doctors and midwives are able to manage these complications effectively before they reach that life-or-death point. In this chapter, we will cover some of the most common complications and even some of those are so uncommon, comparatively speaking, that they barely are worth mentioning.

Malpresentation

Malpresentation simply means that the baby is not in a favorable position for labor and/or delivery. Although the baby can reposition itself during labor, it is more difficult due to the pressure of the contractions restricting fetal movement.

The ideal fetal position for the onset of labor is head down, low in the pelvis. As labor progresses, the baby will rotate so that the face is against the mother's sacrum (lower back) in preparation for the pushing stage.

Breech presentation – In a breech presentation, the butt, butt and feet, or feet are in the pelvis and the head is against the fundus. Babies are breech at the time of active labor approximately 3-4% of the time.

The footling breech is particularly dangerous because once membranes rupture, a foot can pass through a partially dilated cervix and contract cool air, which can cause the baby to take a breath before it is born and aspirate residual amniotic fluid into its lungs.

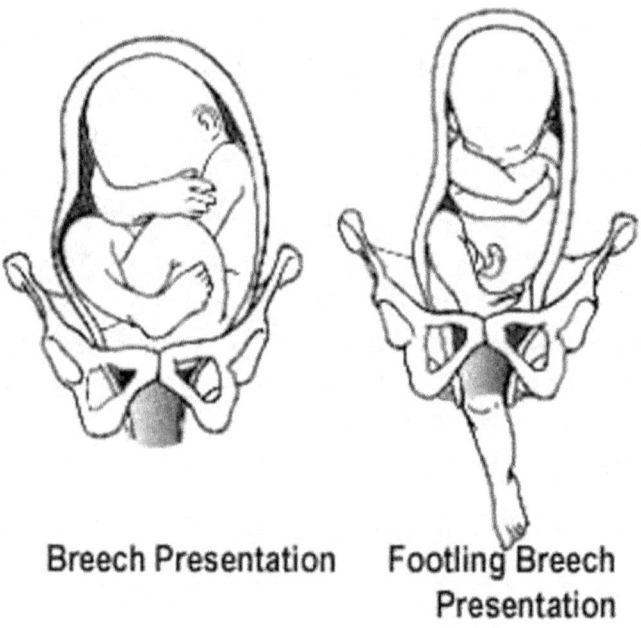

Breech Presentation   Footling Breech Presentation

Breech presentation occurs normally throughout pregnancy as the baby flips and somersaults. The weight of the baby's head as it grows usually forces it into the head down position over time. If the mother is approaching her due date and the baby is still breech, the caregiver may attempt an **external version of breech**.

This is a way of manually manipulating the baby into the correct position:

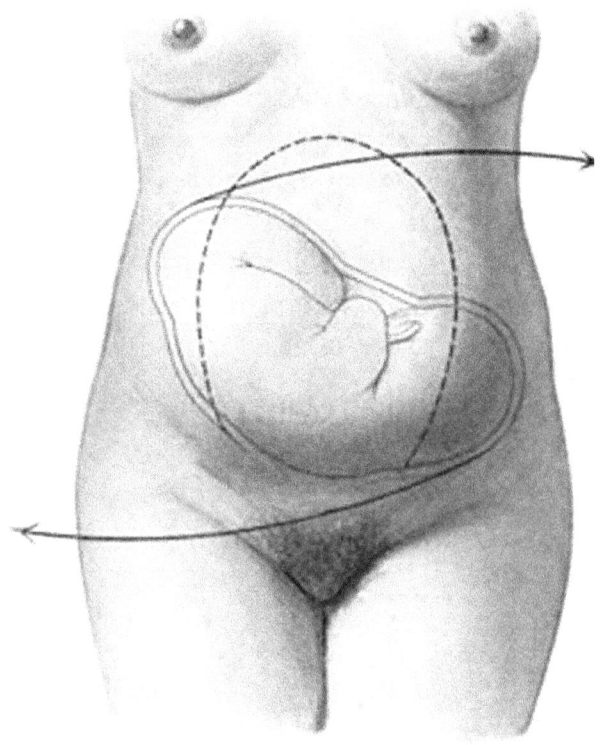

The birth attendant may push, prod, poke, and stroke the baby into a more favorable position in hopes that the much heavier head will keep the baby anchored into the pelvis due to gravity. Sometimes, one of the attendant's hands is inside the mother's vagina, pushing on the lower side of the uterus from within while pushing on the baby from outside on top. This particular maneuver is often quite uncomfortable, as you can imagine.

Another tactic for helping to turn a breech baby is to have the mother get into a knee-chest position with her butt higher than her head for twenty minutes a session, twice a day. Sometimes, this will cause the baby to shift.

It is possible to deliver a breech baby vaginally. The concern, however, is that the smaller, softer body will slip through the mother's pelvis, but the hard, larger head will become stuck. If this happens, the mother will require emergency surgery to have the baby pulled back up through the pelvis. The head of the baby is still inside as the surgery begins and the feet or lower body may be protruding. Exposure to the cooler, outside air is what causes the baby to take its first breath. If the head is still inside and surrounded by residual amniotic fluid and the body is partially exposed, the fear is that the baby will aspirate amniotic fluid into the lungs. Vaginal breech births are more common on a mother who has delivered a baby vaginally before because the pelvis has been "tried."

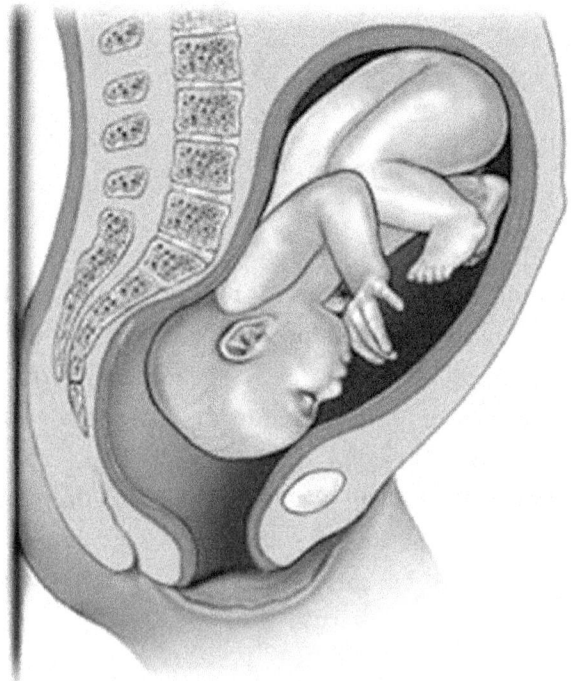

Posterior Presentation – Normally, as the baby emerges from the body, the face is toward the sacrum of the mother's body. Sometimes, the baby faces the pubic bone instead of the sacrum, as seen above.

This is called a posterior presentation, which occurs in approximately 4% of births when the mother does not have an epidural anesthesia and approximately 13% of births when the mother does have an epidural anesthesia. Most babies who are "occiput posterior" will rotate into the correct position as active labor progresses.

The baby can be delivered a posterior presentation, however, the front of the face does not flex as well as the neck when passing under the pubic bone, so pushing may take longer.

Another affect of posterior presentation is that the hard, bony back of the head is against the mother's sacrum instead of the soft, smushy face. This results in bone against bone pain in the mother's back with each contraction. This is in addition to the pain of contractions dilating the cervix.

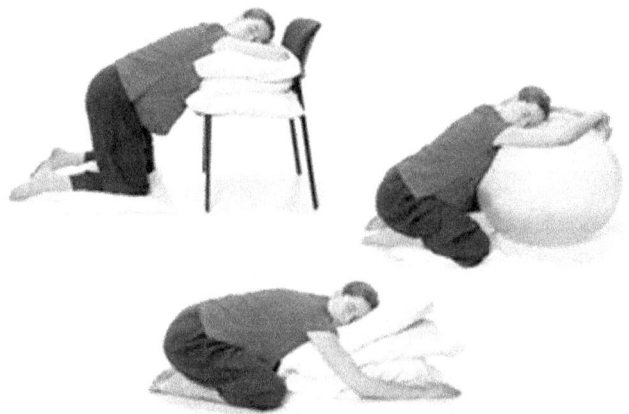

Back labor is very uncomfortable and is treated by postures that allow gravity to pull the baby away from the back, such as those shown in the above illustration. If the laboring mom can perform the "pelvic rock," in which she gets on all fours, tucks in her bottom, then pushes it outward, rocking the pelvis back and forth, this can sometimes turn a posterior baby.

Counter-pressure against the exact point of contact can also be helpful, using the heel of the hand or the tennis balls from the labor bag.

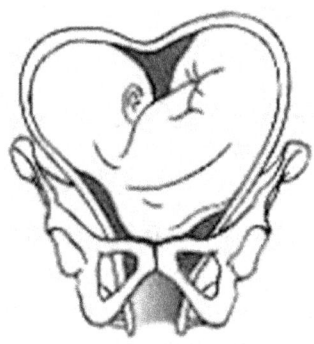

Transverse Lie

Transverse lie – In the transverse presentation, the baby never moves into the pelvis and instead is sideways in the uterus

Not only will the baby be unable to pass through the pelvis in this position, but also there will be no presenting part against the cervix to apply pressure; therefore, it is unlikely that the contractions will produce significant dilation.

Sometimes, a baby in transverse lie can be coaxed into a head down position through external version; however, if this is ineffective, a cesarean will be necessary.

Brow/Face Presentation – In this position, the baby has descended into the pelvis with the brow or the face leading instead of the back of the head. This will make the descent in second stage extremely difficult.

Sometimes, once dilation begins to increase, the caregiver can manually manipulate the baby's head into the correction position. If not, a cesarean is likely.

Maternal or Fetal Distress

One of the common reasons for intervention is when the mother or the baby shows signs of distress either with the pregnancy or the labor and birth. The way the baby tells us of distress is by way of **abnormal fetal heart tones** or by **meconeum staining**. This takes place when the baby has a bowel movement before it is born and the meconeum, the first poop of the baby, is seen in the amniotic fluid, causing it to be green, gray, or brown instead of clear.

Either of these situations is a cause for concern and possibly intervention. For heart tones that are too fast or too slow, the first treatment is to put the mother on her left side and give her supplemental oxygen. Because the majority of blood vessels feeding oxygen to the placenta run up the right side of the body, putting the mother on her left side allows for optimum blood flow of those vessels. Supplemental oxygen to the mother increases the oxygen flow to the baby.

It is normal for the baby's heart tones to decelerate during the contraction, especially after the membranes have ruptured and the amniotic fluid is no longer present to cushion it from the full strength of the contractions. This is not usually cause for concern unless the heart tones are not returning to a healthy level when the contraction ends. This could indicate either that the baby's oxygen in compromised in some way, such as pressure on the umbilical cord, or that there are other reasons why the baby is not withstanding the labor very well.

When the pregnant or laboring woman goes into distress, it is obvious by her demeanor, her words, or her vital signs. She may have an increase in blood pressure that does not change with repositioning. She may spike a fever or show other signs of infection.

In the case of maternal or infant distress, the usual treatment is conservative if possible, escalating to an induction (see below), a cesarean section, or both.

Augmentation and Induction

Augmentation is the attempt to speed up an existing labor. The first means of augmentation is **stripping the membranes**. A caregiver does this during a routine vaginal exam by pushing a finger into the dilated cervix and gently moving the membranes away from the cervix. Stimulation of the membranes can cause the uterus to begin to contract. This process is slightly more uncomfortable than a normal vaginal exam.

The next level of augmentation is to actually rupture the membranes in a procedure called and **amniotomy**. Once the membranes have been ruptured, there is a full commitment to delivery within forty-eight hours due to the risk of infection.

Using an **amniohook,** a plastic hook that resembles a flat crochet hook and has a snagger on the end**...**

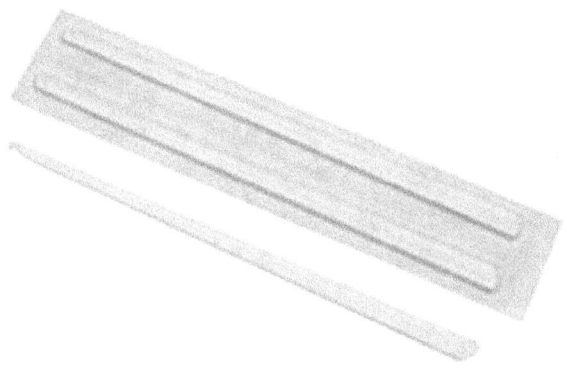

...or an amnicot, a small condom looking sleeve that fits over a finger and has a snagger on the end...

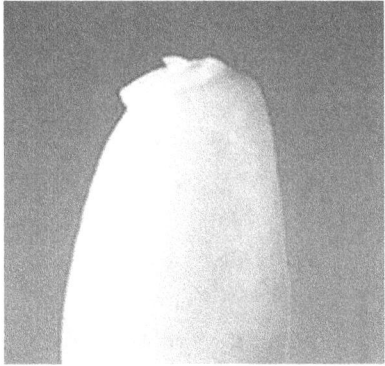

...the caregiver snags the membranes, creating an opening that allows the fluid to leak out.

Ideally, this takes place during active labor while the membranes are bulging through the dilated cervix during a contraction. The cervix must be dilated to allow access to the membranes. Once the water breaks, the head of the baby will make direct contact with the cervix and the labor will move faster. There is merit to leaving the membranes intact for as long as possible as it cushions the baby from the pressure of the contractions and to guard against infection for as long as possible. Once the membranes rupture, there is no longer a barrier between the baby and the outside world.

Another form of augmentation is to give the laboring mother a shot of Pitocin, a synthetic form of the hormone the body releases that causes contraction, to speed up a labor that seems to be losing power as time goes on. This usually goes into her IV.

An **induction of labor** actually initiates labor in a non-laboring woman. In the United States, approximately 22% of labors are induced either for medical purposes or for convenience.

If the woman is slightly dilated, some caregivers will attempt to start labor by breaking the water. This is not the favored way of inducing labor because once the membranes are ruptured, the process is now committed and the baby must be born within forty-eight hours to avoid the risk of infection. The caregiver must be absolutely certain that the mother's body is ready to effectively labor or this practice could result in a domino effect of intervention.

Another way to initiate labor is the use of **prostaglandins**. This involves the insertion of tiny suppositories of prostaglandin material into the cervix during a routine vaginal exam. The prostaglandins look like a string of tiny pearls and dissolve into the cervix, causing it to soften and "ripen" as it releases a contracting agent. This can encourage a labor that is slow to begin to roll over into a successful launch.

The most aggressive form of induction is the use of **Pitocin**, a synthetic form the natural hormone oxytocin, which causes the uterus to contract. A woman is admitted into the hospital and an IV drip is started. When the pitocin is added, this is called a "**pit drip**."

Within approximately twenty minutes, uterine contractions will begin. Induced contractions are extremely intense, beginning at the point of strength and duration as active labor and forcing the uterus to contract aggressively and dilate the cervix. Pitocin inductions are only effective if the uterus is very "ripe" (soft and pliable) and ready to dilate. Elective inductions for the convenience of mother or doctor are now commonplace.

Inductions often open the door for a cesarean section if the induction is unsuccessful and labor is prolonged. The usual reasons for performing an induction will be discussed in the section on Cesarean Sections since inductions and cesarean sections often go hand-in-hand. Women who have an induced labor should prepare for a labor that is much more intense and challenging than a labor that begins spontaneously and is not augmented in any way.

Assisted Birth

An **assisted birth** is the term used when a medical procedure forcefully pulls the baby from the mother's pelvis during the second stage. The two instruments used for this purpose are the **vacuum extractor** and the **forceps:**

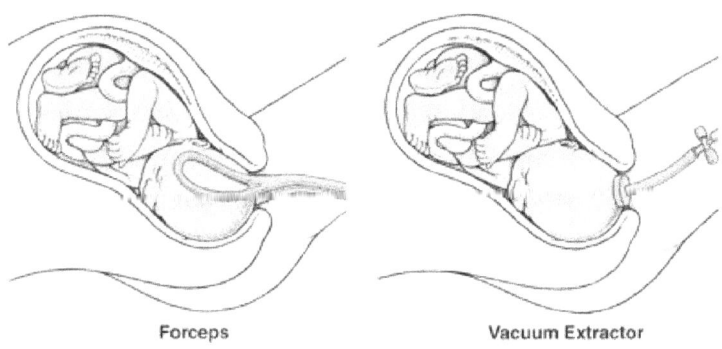

Forceps   Vacuum Extractor

They work pretty much as they appear to work in the picture and should be used only in an emergency to avoid cesarean section. When either is used, a sizeable episiotomy is usually necessary. The vacuum extractor applies focused suction on the baby's head and pulls it out of the vaginal canal and pelvis.

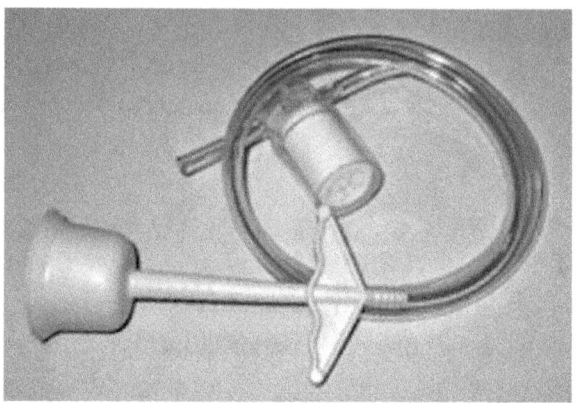

It might look like something Tupperware would sell, but those things are expensive!

The forceps are made of stainless steel and reach up into the uterus or the birth canal to pull the baby down and out. They come apart into two separate blades for easy insertion.

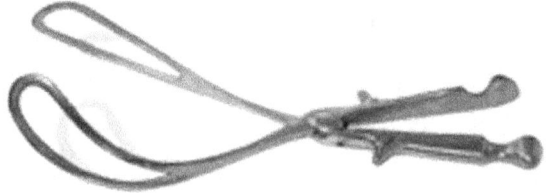

These techniques may be used if the mother is too exhausted from labor and/or prolonged pushing to effectively birth the baby on her own, if the fetal heart tones are very suddenly absent or unfavorable, or if they baby is having difficulty descending through the pelvis.

Another use would be if the baby is malpresenting, such as with a brow or posterior presentation, and the device is used to reposition the baby, then is removed.

Many birth attendants will attempt to first move the baby further into the pelvis by postural treatments such as having the mother squat or get on her knees to push, thereby opening the pelvis more and allowing better shifting of the pelvic bones around the descending baby.

Both the vacuum extractor and forceps can change the way the baby looks when it is born. The baby's skull bones are very soft and pliable at birth, so when the vacuum extractor is used, the head can mold to the shape of the suction cup or leave a bruise mark. Forceps can leave bruises on the baby's cheeks or head.

Other Complications

Premature birth – In a premature birth, labor begins prior to thirty-eight weeks. The viability of the baby will be determined and the caregiver will determine whether to allow the labor to continue or attempt to stop it. If the decision is to stop the labor, the usual treatment is an IV of magnesium sulfate and bed rest. This may or may not work. Premature infants have significantly greater health challenges than term babies. Any baby weighing less than 5 pounds, 8 ounces is considered "low birth weight." Of course, the longer a baby remains in the uterus, the better, since the finishing touches on vital organs, especially the kidneys, are very important. Low birth weight infants carry a huge risk for many ailments.

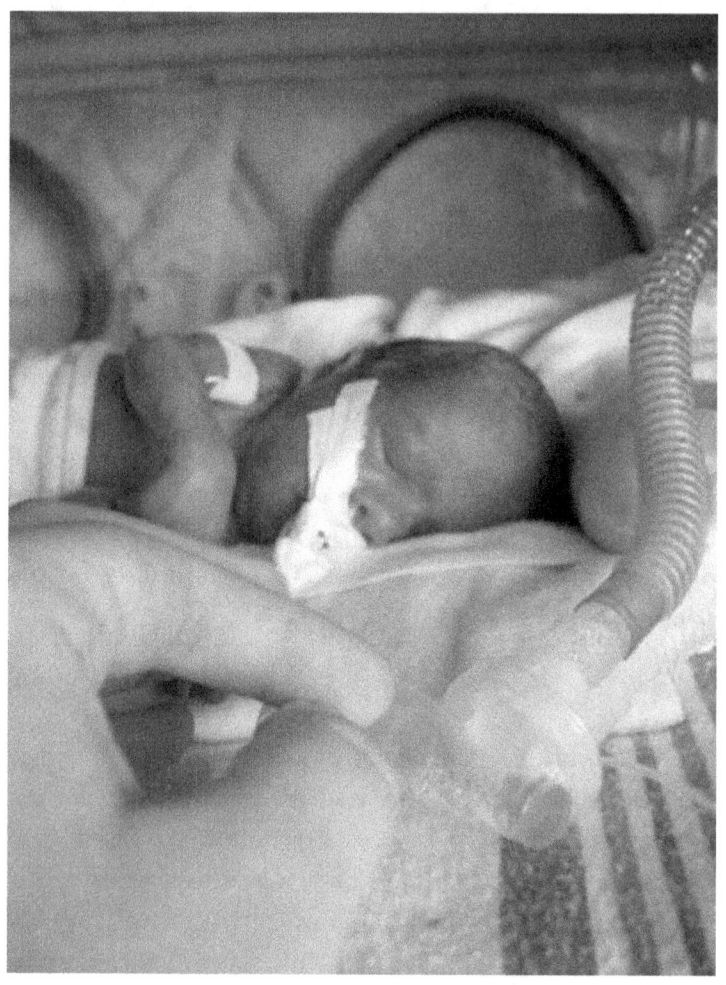

Maternal hemorrhage – If the uterus does not properly "clamp down" on the placental wound after stage 3 of labor, the mother may hemorrhage or "bleed out." This can lead to a condition called **hypovolemic shock.** This condition is usually quickly managed with drugs such as Pitocin or methergine, aggressive uterine massage, nipple stimulation or breastfeeding, and if necessary, transfusion protocol.

Cesarean Section

A **cesarean section** is the surgical removal of the baby through the mother's abdominal wall. Because it involves an incision into the abdominal way, it is considered a major surgery and the recovery period is much longer than for a routine vaginal birth.

There is a rumor that the cesarean section got its name because Julius Caesar was delivered in this manner. At the time of Caeser's birth, pregnant women did not survive the procedure and Caesar's mother was known to live for quite some time after his birth, so this myth is busted. There is no record of a woman surviving a c-section prior to 1500 AD.

The actual name comes, as do so many medical terms, from the Latin language. The word *"caedere"* means *"to cut"* and is thought to provide the etymology of the word.

The rule used to be "once a cesarean, always a cesarean," but the past several decades perfected the practice of the VBAC (Vaginal Birth After Cesarean) as long as the reason for the original cesarean is not present for the current birth. A pregnant woman can usually elect to have a repeat cesarean rather than a VBAC if that is her choice.

Most women are now awake for their cesarean sections, choosing an epidural anesthesia in order to be present for their baby's first moments in the outside world. Unless there is a dire emergency necessitating the surgery, a support person can usually be with the woman.

The cesarean section field is set up in such a way that a screen is up between the mother's shoulders and the rest of her body. She will see the baby being lifted up and may have a few minutes to bond.

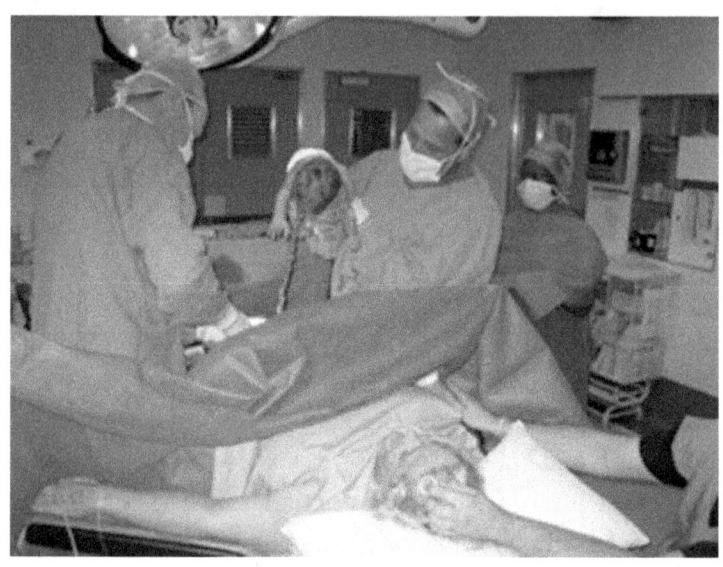

Most babies born by cesarean section require extensive suctioning to remove mucus from their respiratory tract. Normally, this mucus gets pushed out of the lungs and windpipe by the pressure of moving through the birth canal.

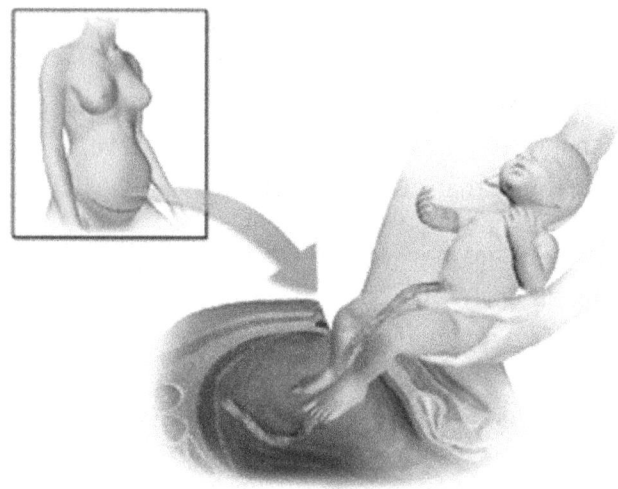

In the case of a cesarean section, a horizontal incision is made just above the pubic bone. The uterus is then incised just above the cervix. The surgeon inserts a hand into the uterus to disengage the baby's head from the pelvis while pressure is put on the fundus. The baby is delivered through the incision with the placenta and membranes following shortly afterward, having also been manually removed.

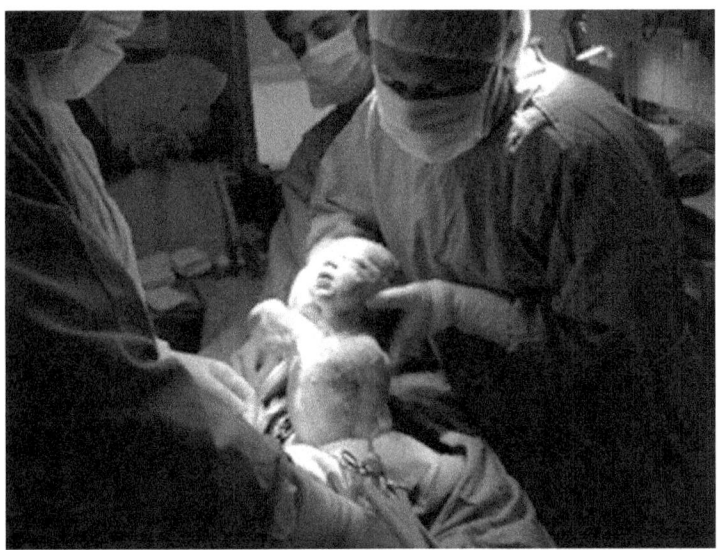

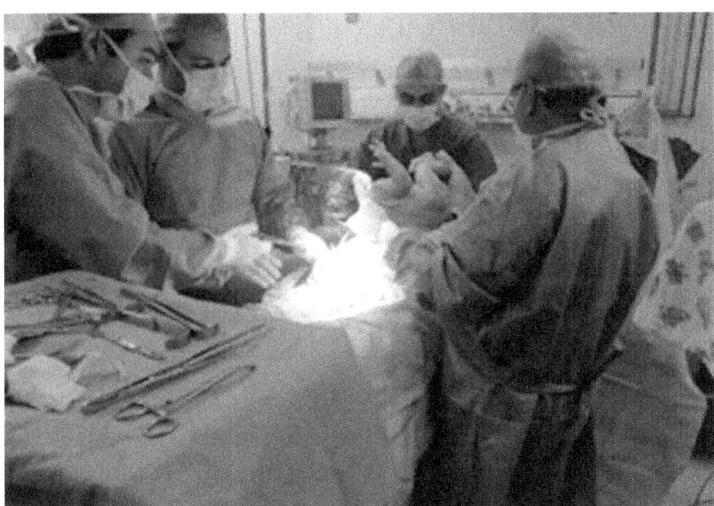

After the placenta and membranes are removed, the uterus and abdominal wall are repaired and the outer layer of skin is secured with staples. The scar will often be nearly invisible in the natural folds of the skin.

Staples are removed within a few days of the surgery with a special staple removing tool. Stitches dissolve without a need for removal.

Possible reasons for an induction or cesarean section or both include:

Toxemia/pre-eclampsia – These are very similar conditions that result in rising blood pressure and an inability to absorb protein. It is characterized by extreme water retention and swelling (edema), plus a higher level of protein in the urine. Initial treatment involves bed rest and increased water intake. If the blood pressure does not normalize, the labor may need to be artificially induced. If the induction is not effective, a cesarean section may be required. This condition begins to resolve as soon as the baby is born.

Chorioamnionitis – This is an infection of the chorion, the outer amniotic membrane. It is rare and characterized by maternal fever and uterine tenderness. This condition occurs when the membranes rupture and bacteria contaminate the uterine environment through the vaginal canal. When signs of chorioamnionitis present, the baby needs to be delivered as soon as possible. Depending on the severity of the infection, an induction or cesarean may be performed.

Failure to Progress or Failure to Descend – With *failure to progress*, there is insufficient dilation for the delivery to occur. *Failure to descend* means that the pushing stage is prolonged and the baby is not making adequate progress through the pelvis and birth canal. A prolonged labor in either the first or second stage can be challenging for both the mother and the baby and it is critical that their condition be monitored carefully should this occur.

One reason for failure to descend is a condition known as cephalopelvic disproportion (CPD), meaning the head is too big to fit through the pelvis. This condition is not normally diagnosed until prolonged pushing without sufficient progress has occurred.

Another reason could involve a very long umbilical cord that is twined around the baby's body in such a way that descent into and through the pelvis is not possible. This circumstance is usually indicated by poor heart tones during labor or pushing and failure of the baby to move through the pelvis. It is normally not confirmed until cesarean section when the surgeon sees the cord around the baby.

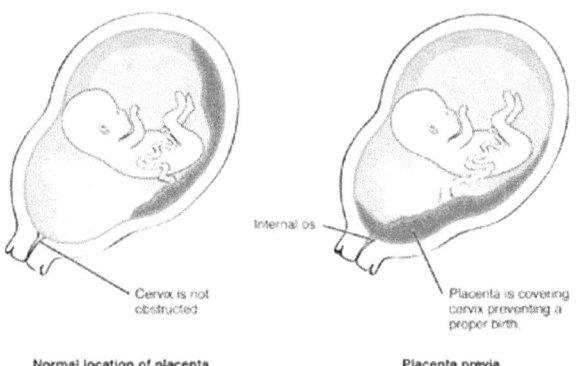

Normal location of placenta   Placenta previa

Placenta Previa – Very rarely, during the time of conception and the subsequent weeks, the placenta attaches over the opening of the cervix rather than onto the uterine wall. This creates a physical barrier to the baby's exit from the uterus and a danger of hemorrhage to both mother and baby since the placenta will begin separate as even the earliest dilation begins.

This condition will usually be detected by an early sonogram. A cesarean section will be scheduled before the mother goes into labor to avoid dilation beginning. If the condition is not seen by sonogram, the first indication of placenta previa is bright red bleeding from the vagina, indicating that separation of the placenta has begun. This would be an emergency cesarean situation as both the mother and the baby are bleeding out from the separation site.

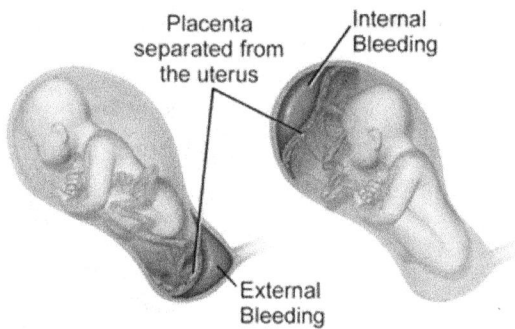

Abruptio Placenta (Placental Abruption)

Placental Abruption – An abruption occurs when the placenta begins to separate from the wall of the uterus before the baby is born. As the placenta separates, not only does bleeding occur between the membranes and the wall of the uterus, but also the baby's oxygen supply is diminished due to the placenta's failure to make full contact with the uterus. The most common cause of an abruption is extreme postmaturity. The placenta has a finite lifespan, usually around forty-two weeks, and once that is passed, it begins to calcify around the edges and deteriorate. This is the primary reason that caregivers become concerned about a pregnancy that goes beyond the forty week point. An abruption is characterized by vaginal bleeding and extreme rigidity of the uterine wall.

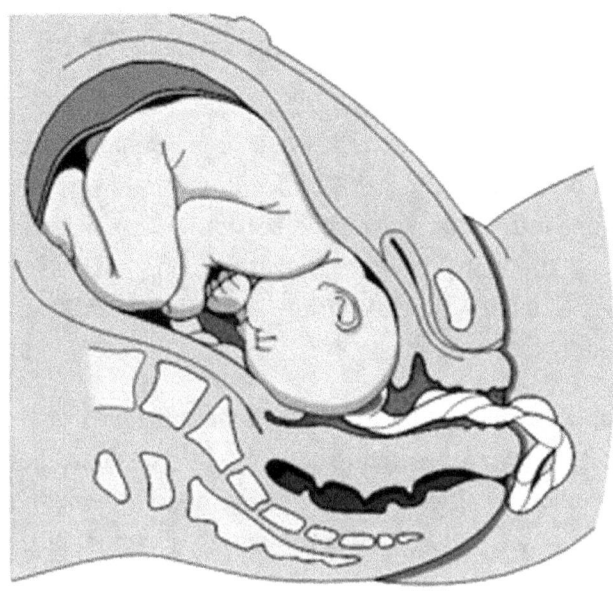

Umbilical cord prolapse – This condition takes place primarily when the baby's head is not well engaged into the pelvis and the membranes rupture prematurely. The cord washes down into the vagina ahead of the baby. The risk is that the cord will contract fresh air and the Wharton's jelly will activate, causing the cord to contract and cut off blood supply to the baby before birth occurs.

This is a matter of extreme danger to the baby. If the mother feels the cord in the vagina, she should immediately assume a knee chest position to allow gravity to pull the cord as close to the baby as possible. The mother should then be transported without delay *in that position* to the nearest hospital for an emergency cesarean section.

Gestational Diabetes – If the mother has gestational diabetes, she has a tendency to have a larger-than-usual baby due to the high sugar levels in her bloodstream. Some caregivers will induce labor to allow for delivery of the baby not only to end the gestational diabetes, but also to prevent cephalopelvic disproportion due to the increasing size of the baby.

Active Herpes Outbreak – If the mother is experiencing an active outbreak of Herpes Simplex II (vaginal herpes) when she goes into labor, a cesarean section will be necessary to prevent the baby from passing the skin that has active herpes lesions. Although herpes is painful to adults, it can be deadly to newborns.

Multiple Births – A mother who is having twins or triplets will often have a cesarean section if all babies are not in a head down position. If babies are head down and the largest baby is engaged into the pelvis, a vaginal birth may be possible. If the both babies are not head down, most caregivers will opt for a cesarean section due to the breech birth risk. If the largest baby is head down, some caregivers will allow a vaginal birth knowing that if the larger baby fit through the pelvis, the smaller breech baby will as well.

The Spiritual Aspect of Birth Complications

It is extremely frustrating and frightening when a birth does not go as you imagined and moms often have to go through a long adjustment period to reconcile that the birth they dreamed of and planned did not happen. Feelings of failure and disappointment are very common when birth requires major intervention of some kind.

There are many platitudes that all make perfect sense in this situation. "It is what it is." "You have to trust the process." "Be thankful the medical staff was there." "There's always next time." "At least you have a healthy baby." Nothing anyone says to you can really make it better until you are ready to move beyond what has happened.

Some people take birth complications harder than others. The healthy approach, of course, is to say, "You know, we did all we could do and the resources were there when we needed them." By the numbers, birth complications are rare, but when they do happen, their impact is very individual. The laboring woman who faces a crisis must trust in her support team to help her make wise choices. To do this, everyone involved must be educated about the birthing process and hospital procedures, but also must trust their instincts as well.

I have had women call me crying about cesarean sections tearfully confessing to me that they "failed" at prepared childbirth. I have had others say the same thing because in the intensity of birth, they chose to have an epidural instead of "toughing it out."

Each woman has their own experience and *there is no failure*. Going into any labor, there is no way of knowing what a woman will need in order to work with her body in the best way possible. We can take plenty of notes and create the finest birth plan ever, but until those contractions are really taking hold, we truly have no idea how we will react or what our bodies will need.

You always simply do the best you can do. I have had six children. For five of those births, I received no medication at all. I am profoundly grateful for those experiences, but I know that if I ever faced childbirth again, it is possible I would make very different choices. I knew that going into each of my births.

CHAPTER 12 – EMERGENCY BIRTH

One of the most dramatic experiences for a pregnant woman and her support team is for labor to advance so quickly that she must give birth away from her safe and planned environment.

What is the first thing you hear on television or in the movies when a woman is about to give birth unexpectedly? "Boil hot water!" The only thing you will need hot water for in the case of emergency childbirth is to make tea to help everyone around her relax. Most people immediately think of using boiling water to disinfect instruments that will be used in the birth. The fact is that when emergency childbirth is done correctly and safely, no instruments will be needed.

Can you imagine the most common place where women give birth unexpectedly? It is actually in the parking lot of a hospital. Many start driving and realize the labor is more advanced than they thought it was, drive as far as the hospital and then are unable to get the mom to move from the vehicle.

During my career with birth, which spanned a little less than twenty years, I knew of several incidents where parents delivered their own babies without the assistance of medical staff. One couple started driving, realized the baby coming out and delivered in the back of their van. There is now a woman in her early 30s named "Chevy" as a result.

Another student of mine felt a low backache through the day that intensified enough to wake her up after a few hours of sleeping. She thought she might be constipated and went to the bathroom. After urinating, she wiped and felt the baby's head at the vaginal opening. Within minutes, she was holding a perfectly healthy baby boy.

Fortunately, in each of these situations, the couples were taught exactly what to do if they found themselves in this very circumstance.

Most people believe panic would take over, but almost universally, the panic comes later, after the birth has taken place, as they realize the enormity of what just happened. At the time, the pregnant mom and those around her become very intent on taking care of the immediate crisis.

It helps to remember that women labored and delivered without medical staff for thousands of years. It is also reassuring to know that if the baby is coming so fast that you cannot get to a medical facility, there is likely very little holding it back such as the umbilical cord wrapped around the body, malpresentation, or a tight fit through the pelvis. For things to proceed this quickly, there is a very clear and safe path right to the outside world. Rarely do medical complications of labor and delivery take place when the baby is being born precipitously.

The most common scenario for this circumstance is that the water breaks and contractions begin quickly. Some women will by-pass the preliminary stage and go right into active labor with contractions that are only two to three minutes apart. When the mother realizes labor is beginning, she likely thinks she is experiencing early labor. On very rare occasions, the situations are perfect for a very quick delivery: no obstacles, very relaxed mom with a high pain threshold, very soft, "ripe" cervix and vaginal tissues, and a motivated baby.

If the mother is not feeling an urge to bear down or can fight the urge if she is feeling it, transportation to the hospital or place of birth should continue. The mother should be encouraged to blow forcefully through her mouth during the contractions to avoid pushing and moving the baby down faster. **The driver should continue toward the destination unless and until the words are spoken (or shouted), "*I can feel the baby coming.*"**

When the mother states that she can feel the baby moving downward and into the vaginal canal, the transportation should stop. If cell service is available, **call an ambulance** immediately. If anyone stops to help, tell him or her to get an ambulance right away if one is not already on the way. Whatever you do, *stay with the laboring mother!*

The first job of the newly appointed birth attendant is to get the mother as comfortable as possible. Jackets, pillows, bags, or whatever is handy should be used to prop her up into a comfortable position for delivery, making certain the attendant has access to her vaginal area. A person needs a little elbowroom around them to catch the baby.

The mother should be encouraged to relax as much as possible. It is essential that the attendant look and act as though they are in control and calm, even if that is not how they feel on the inside. The mother is very vulnerable to suggestion at this point in her labor. If someone looks directly at her, makes eye contact, and says, "You and your baby are going to be just fine, but I need for you to do exactly what I tell you to do," it is likely she will believe them and focus on the task of birthing. If the attendant is scattered and in a panic, she will notice this energy quickly and panic herself, which will deprive the baby of much-needed oxygen and create tension.

The mother should continue to blow through the contractions. If she pushes with the baby already coming this fast, she could tear her vaginal tissues. The baby will be born through the strength of the contractions alone.

It is possible that the mother feels the baby moving downward, but the attendant does not yet see anything. The attendant should begin to massage the vaginal opening very gently to prepare it for the baby's descent. If several minutes pass and there is no sign of the baby, the attendant should get the mother settled and start driving again.

If, however, the attendant sees the baby's head starting to come down, he or she should gently work the vaginal tissues over and behind it as it begins to crown. The vaginal tissues should not be allowed to extend over the baby's head like a cap or the mother may tear.

IMPORTANT: At no time should the attendant or the mother attempt to push the baby upward into the birth canal or hold the mother's legs together to prevent birth. This can create extremely dangerous circumstances for the baby.

It is normal for the head to look misshapened as it emerges. The skull bones of the cranium overlap one another at the suture line that runs between the two fontanelles. This will resolve as soon as the head is free of the pressure of the birth canal and the head will round out again, so *do not panic* if you see something very alien coming out.

When the head crowns, the mother will likely gasp and pull back as she feels the stinging, burning sensation called the "ring of fire." The sensation is over almost as soon as it begins and from that point until after the baby is out, the mother's vaginal opening will be numb.

The attendant should continue to massage the skin back. It is normal for there to be some mild bleeding from capillary rupture in the cervix. As the head emerges, it will likely face downward. The head will duck under the pubic bone and flex upward as it emerges. The attendant should attempt to gently squeeze the baby's nose to push out any mucus that may have collected in the nostrils.

On the next contraction, the head will begin to rotate in the attendant's hands. This occurs because the body is rotating inside the mother in order to birth the shoulders through the pelvic opening. When the head begins to turn, the attendant should immediately grab a cloth of some kind (the most commonly used item is their own shirt) and hold it over their hands. This will provide traction to grab the baby as it emerges.

Do not kid yourself. Once the head has turned and the upper shoulder is born, the baby is going to shoot out of the vaginal opening under the pressure of the contraction. The baby is covered in amniotic fluid which is very alkaline and therefore, very slippery. The attendant should BE PREPARED and NOT DROP THIS BABY! The shirt is more valuable than I can express at aiding in the catch. A thin towel also works well if one is available.

As the baby exits, the mother will likely relax immediately from exhaustion. The attendant should make certain she is relaxing and not passing out. Talk to her. She should be breathing normally now and is likely quite anxious.

The immediate concern is to get the baby breathing. If the birth occurs in an outside environment, even in a car, the cooler air will likely startle the baby into a cry. If a baby is crying, a baby is breathing. If the baby is not breathing, the attendant should turn the baby over along their forearm with the forearm lower than the elbow so the head is pointed downward, then gently but firmly massage and pat the baby's back to attempt to dislodge any mucus that may be trapped in the throat. They should also run a pinky finger around the inside of the baby's mouth to remove any residual mucus from the mouth.

If the baby does not begin to breathe, the attendant may also turn the baby over on its back along the forearm and gently stroke the line from the baby's breastbone up the throat, again to attempt to dislodge any remaining mucus. The attendant can rub the baby's cheeks, talk to the baby, and if necessary, flick the bottoms of the baby's feet to help it to wake up and start breathing. A precipitous birth like this is so rigorous that most babies born in emergency births come out howling.

This sounds scary, but it is important to note that this situation is not as critical as it appears. While the placenta is still attached, the baby continues to receive oxygen through the umbilical cord. The cord has been exposed to air and will quickly begin to contract down on itself and cut off the blood flow, but you have several minutes before the oxygen is completely cut off. Again, it is rare that a baby involved in an emergency birth is not crying due to the hyperstimulation of a quick birth.

Once it is established that the baby is breathing, the baby should quickly be put to the breast regardless of whether or not the mother intended to breastfeed. Nursing at this time will stimulate oxytocin to release, which will allow for a clean separation of the placenta and help prevent hemorrhage of the mother from the placental wound site after separation.

The mother should hold the baby to her breast, naked skin against naked skin, and tickle the side of the baby's mouth with the nipple of the breast. The baby will then root around to look for the breast. The mother should then push as much of her nipple and areola into the baby's open mouth as possible and wait for the baby to latch on and start to nurse.

Meanwhile, the attendant now needs to wait and catch the placenta. As the placenta separates, there will be a rush of blood from the vagina. At that time, the mother should use one hand to push into her abdomen until she finds her uterus, which is now about the size of a football. She should use her fist or the heel of her hand to push into the uterus firmly and repeatedly to cause it to contract down onto the placental wound site. This is a kneading action, like a massage. The placenta will sort of plop off out of the vagina. Yes, the attendant must catch it because the hospital staff will want to inspect it.

The baby should be placed in the cloth the attendant used to catch it and the cord and placenta should be piled onto the baby's groin area. The entire package of baby and afterbirth should then be wrapped in the cloth and the baby returned immediately to the breast with as much skin-to-skin contact with the mother as possible. If no emergency response team is on site by the time the baby is wrapped and the mother is stable, the attendant should drive the mother and baby to the Emergency Room.

Please notice that at NO TIME was the instruction present to cut the umbilical cord. Medical staff will want to inspect the placenta for missing pieces and to check the umbilical cord. Cutting the cord leads to a potential for hemorrhage and infection. The back of the placenta may seep blood slightly, but the blood transfer between the baby and the placenta ceases once the Wharton's jelly takes effect and the cord begins to compress shortly after birth.

CHAPTER 13 – IN CONCLUSION

In a perfect world, every woman would give birth in exactly the way she chooses. There would be no fertility struggles. We would conceive every baby in love and ecstasy then welcome them into a stable family with no financial or emotional concerns. Every mother would be in touch with her baby from the beginning and glow with the beauty of pregnancy, then deliver surrounded by the people who make her feel safest and most loved.

In absence of that perfection, it falls to us to create our birthing experience by managing it in the way that are available to us. For an increasing number of women, that includes connecting to their pregnancy and their baby in a meaningful way and bringing the power of the Divine, whether that be God, Goddess, Creator, The Universe, or whatever label is assigned.

All religions that I know of see nature as an expression of Divine energy. Little is more natural than the birth process that furthers the species and continually evolves us to the next level and by those standards, birth is already a divine process. Tapping into the your own body's magnificent and phenomenal capabilities to carry and birth a baby is a profoundly spiritual process when you trust yourself, educate yourself, and do the homework to create the birth plan you want to follow. Choose your caregiver with tremendous thought and be certain that they support your birthing ambitions and will act with you and your baby's best interests in focus rather than the routine procedures that attempt to standardize an experience as individual as birth.

As carefully as you choose your attendants, assemble the support team that helps you to feel empowered and protected and above all, around whom you can be yourself without reservation. Imagine that you are creating the team with whom you will take on the Zombie Apocalypse. Who has your back? Who can calmly manage a crisis? Who is not going to flake and run when things get rough? Who will allow you to both surrender and be strong without feeling threatened? Who is not going to let petty, emotional crap get in the way of the important stuff?

Create your birth fortress of information, preparation, and support, so that you can comfortably relax, tune into your body and what it is doing, connect with your baby to work as a team, and feel the power of the Divine course through you. As I pointed out earlier in this book, for most women, childbirth only happens a few times in their lives. When it happens to you, recognize that there are often more choices available than you immediately see. Be gentle with yourself and dare to imagine how you want your birthing experience to be. Use that vision to craft the birth that is right for you and allow no one, not even me, tell you how it should be.

Blessings to you and your baby.

APPENDIX 1 – BREATHING TECHNIQUES

One of the activities most associated with prepared childbirth classes other than walking into a room of strangers carrying armloads of pillows is breathing in odd ways. Once again, television and movies get it wrong and portray fast, intense breathing.

The goal of breathing through contractions is twofold. It is human tendency to tense up when we are in pain and to roll up into a ball when we have abdominal pain. The main discomfort from labor contractions tends to be in the lower abdomen where the cervix is opening to allow the baby to be born. The natural tendency to curl into a ball with abdominal pain usually makes perfect sense because it uses our body to protect the vulnerable area. Unfortunately, when we give over to those natural urges specifically in labor, the larger muscle groups, arms, legs, abdominal muscles, and lateral muscles, all close in on the uterus, which is trying to contract to open the cervix. Imagine if you make a fist and try to open it while someone closes their larger hand over the fist you are trying to open.

In order to allow the uterus to contract without interference from surrounding muscle groups, the laboring mother must remain very relaxed and distracted from any pain or discomfort she feels. Because the uterus is an extremely muscular organ and is working very hard, it requires huge amounts of oxygen. Another natural response to pain is to hold one's breath. Unfortunately, this cuts off the flow of oxygen to both the uterus and to the baby, who undergoes stress during the labor contractions, especially after the membranes rupture and the amniotic fluid is no longer present as a buffer.

Using patterned breathing techniques not only distracts the mother from any pain she is feeling by allowing her to focus on her breathing, but it also keeps a steady flow of oxygen going to the uterus and to the baby during the contraction.

It is sometimes helpful for the woman's partner to do the breathing with her during labor to help her to stay on track and maintain the breathing pattern. This is why it is important for both the pregnant woman and her support person to learn and practice the breathing techniques.

There are four breathing techniques that most laboring women helpful. Each one should be practiced frequently because the technique a woman favors when she is not in labor may not be the most effective when she is in labor.

Cleansing breath – This is a very deep breath in the nose and out the mouth taken as the contraction begins and as it ends. It signals the support person that another contraction is coming and gives the baby and the uterus a big boost of oxygen before and after the contraction. The cleansing breath is drawn in the nose for a count of four and exhaled through the mouth for a count of four.

Slow chest breathing – This is similar to the cleansing breath, but is not quite as deep. It is a slowing down of regular breathing. The cleansing breath is audible, but the slow chest breathing is very quiet. Simply breathe in the nose for a count of four and exhale through the mouth for a count of four. Some women are able to use slow chest breathing throughout the entire labor process.

Panting – This type of breathing is adapted from the breathing of animals when they labor and is very effective. As labor progresses, the uterus begins to experience muscle fatigue and becomes sore like any other muscle that is overworked. When the laboring woman breathes deeply, such as with slow chest breathing, the lungs expand, which pushes the diaphragm against the contracting uterus. It is possible that the uterus will become intolerant of the pressure of the movement of the diaphragm against it. This manifests in the form of increased uterine pain.

If the laboring mother finds that slow chest breathing in no longer effectively keeping her distracted, she can switch to panting.

Panting is done by bringing the breathing up higher in the chest and making it very light. She should breathe in and out of the mouth and on the exhale, make the sound "Heeeee." The inhale sounds like "Ahhh." It almost feels as though she is taking a short breath in and blowing the same breath out again. This breathing is very light and quiet.

As breathing speeds up for the panting, the nasal passages would dry out if she did not move breathing to in and out the mouth. She should pant as slowly as she can and still remain in control during the contraction.

Pant-Blow – As labor progresses, some people need more distraction to remain in control. By incorporating a gentle "blow" into the breathing pattern, the laboring woman has to think more about maintaining the pattern, which creates greater distraction.

The blow part of the pattern is no stronger than the panting. The mouth is simply reshaped from a "hee" to a "blow."

The pattern might be a three-pant blow pattern:

Ah hee, ah hee, ah hee, ah blow, ah hee, ah hee, ah hee, ah blow...

…or a two pant blow:

Ah hee, ah hee, ah blow, ah hee, ah hee, ah blow…

…or a one-pant blow:

Ah hee, ah blow, ah hee, ah blow, ah hee, ah blow…

The more frequently the blow is incorporated into the breathing pattern, the greater the distraction. As the breathing patterns speed up, the laboring mother should keep her effleurage (rubbing the tummy with big, soft circles) slow, again, increasing the distraction.

As labor intensifies, the mom may want to mix her breathing techniques, using slow chest breathing to start, then moving on to panting, then to pant blow, then back to panting and ending with slow chest breathing all in one contraction. This keeps her attuned to the rise and fall of the contraction.

The mother should keep her breathing in the lowest level she can and still remain comfortable. The higher the level of breathing, the greater the risk of hyperventilation.

APPENDIX 2 – THE BAGGAGE

Any **admission forms** your facility requires.

A **baby name book** in case you have not yet decided

A **camera or video camera** with **extra batteries** and **storage space**. Do not presume that there will be a place to charge your phone or camera in the labor area.

Cell phone

Lunch-sized paper bag in case she hyperventilates. If she begins to get light-headed, the support person should have her breathe into the paper bag, continuing her usual breathing techniques.

Cash for food or the vending machines

Insurance information

A **book** like this one for reference in case something weird comes up.

Two tennis balls in a sock for a back massage tool. Tennis balls give great counter pressure to the specific part of the back getting pressure from the inside. If you keep them in a sock with the open end tied closed, they will not get away from you in the labor room.

Washcloth from home, colored so that it does not get swept away with the hospital laundry. The washcloth is great for putting cool cloths on the laboring woman's forehead, chest, or the back of the neck. In fact, bring a couple of them. You can also wet the washcloth with cool water and wrap it around ice chips to give her something to wet her lips as she labors.

Tupperware rolling pin – The big thing about a Tupperware rolling pin is that it is plastic and hollow, so you can fill it with hot water. This makes a great tool for back massage or to use as a hot water bottle against her lower abdomen.

Copy of your **birth plan** for your labor staff to see.

Suckers, sour preferred – Suckers are instant energy due to their sugar content and sour suckers will cause the mouth to produce more saliva. Dry mouth can be a problem in labor and suckers will help lubricate the mouth. Do not bring hard candies that are not on a stick because it is challenging to fish around in your mouth for a candy when a contraction comes on suddenly and you need to breathe. Labor contractions are a lot less fun when someone is performing the Heimlich maneuver on you.

Unscented lotion for massage – self explanatory. Scents often cause women to wretch in labor, so unscented.

Watch or clock with a second hand or readout for timing contractions and secondarily, for keeping track of time because it is easy to get disoriented in labor and have no idea how long you have been there or in labor.

Focal Point – Keeping your eyes focused on one places helps to externalize yourself away from the pain of contractions. When you practice your breathing techniques (see Appendix 1) pick a portable item you can use for a focal point and then take it with you to your birthing place. This gives you a sense of the familiar that can be comforting.

Books/magazines/reading device

Extra pillows – You can never have enough

FOOD - small cooler or non-perishable items that do NOT have a strong smell. Even though the laboring woman is usually not very hungry, support people feel as though they will starve when labor goes on for hours. Because strong smells can cause a laboring woman to vomit, leave the onions, Slim Jims, Snickers, and other smelly snacks at home.

Thick socks – When a woman labors, her blood supply centralizes in her abdomen to nourish the contracting uterus. This causes her feet to get cold.

Something to tie back your hair – If there is any chance that the laboring woman's hair or a support person's hair will get in their face, you have to be able to tie it back. If you are sitting up in bed, having your hair tied up on the back of your head will be annoying. Ponytails usually work best.

Unscented lip balm – Again with the dry mouth, spreading to dry, cracked lips.

Mouthwash/breath mints – Both laboring woman and support staff can get buffalo breath after breathing in and out the mouth for hours.

Suitcase

Address Book/contact list

Baby Book (get the staff to footprint the baby)

Thank you cards/notes

Large bag to bring home gifts and hospital supplies

Clothing to wear home

Bathrobe

Loose, comfortable outfits for hospital stay

Nightgown

Nursing bras

Nursing pads

Slippers

Underwear

Personal toiletries

Earplugs and Eye mask – it can be busy at night.

Glasses if needed

Maxipads – biggest ones you can find

Prescription medications you're taking

Approved car seat

Diapers for the trip home

Going-home outfit

Hat/cap

Receiving blankets

APPENDIX 3 – PROGRESSION OF A LABOR CONTRACTION

- Laboring mother feels the contraction begin

- Deep cleansing breath in the nose and out the mouth

- Lock onto focal point on the exhalation of the cleansing breath and do not look away from it for the duration of the contraction (usually 60-90 seconds). Later in labor, the support person's eyes make a great focal point.

- Immediately after the exhalation, begin patterned breathing (slow chest, panting, pant-blow, or a modified technique) and effleurage (very lightly rubbing the belly with large circles – this is performed by the laboring mother to increase distraction and block the pain sensation)

- Mother actively relaxes all parts of her body.

- Support person gently checks her body for tension using touch and sight. Pay close attention to shoulders, jaw, and hands. If the support person detects tension, they say, "Relax your ___," very softly, gently touching the area.

- Mother continues to maintain her focal point, relax her entire body around the contracting uterus, and using her patterned breathing techniques, shifting to a more intense breathing technique if needed as the strength of the contraction builds.

- Mother slows down the patterned breathing as the contraction lessens in strength.

- Cleansing breath as the contraction ends.

- Between contractions, mother conveys to the support person anything she needs and support person works to help her become comfortable, using supplies from the labor bag, position changes, more pillows, or whatever she needs.

The mother's pain relief measures are all dedicated to the goal of relaxation. As pain increases, the more she is distracted from the pain, the better she is able to relax around the contracting uterus so it can do its job effectively.

APPENDIX 4 – NON-MEDICATION PAIN RELIEF MEASURES FOR LABOR

- Support person using voice and touch to assist with relaxation

- Pillows, chairs, labor bed adjustments, and other items to create a comfortable position during each contraction

- Items from the Labor Bag to increase comfort

- Warm towels, cool washcloths

- Swaying, vocalizing or humming (one woman I knew sang show tunes until she was pushing)

- Cleansing breaths

- Patterned breathing techniques

- Focal point

- Effleurage

- Eye-to-eye contact during breathing

- Visualization of the body opening to release the baby ("open and release" or "down and out" thoughts)

-Squatting, frequent posture changes

- Birthing ball

- Warm baths or water birth

ABOUT THE AUTHOR

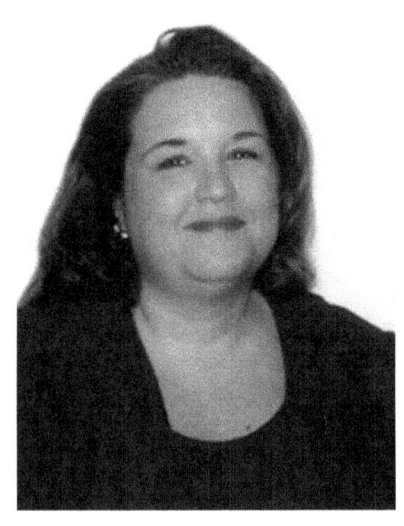

Katrina Rasbold is a prolific published author and journalist. She taught prepared childbirth classes and early pregnancy classes from 1980-1997 and apprenticed as a midwife in New Mexico. She worked as a doula and continues to work as a childbirth instructor. Her work in the field of adult education is varied and currently, she teaches workshop on Women's Mysteries and techniques of energy manipulation for positive manifestation. Katrina has a PhD in Religion with a minor in Psychology and is the owner of Rasbold Ink. She has been an online publisher since 2000. Her books can be found at www.katrinarasbold.com. She may also be booked for personal appearances at that same website

OTHER BOOKS BY THE AUTHOR

Energy Magic

Energy Magic Compleat

Beyond Energy Magic

The CUSP Way

Properties of Magical Energy

Reuniting the Two Selves

Magical Ethics and Protection

The Art of Ritual Crafting

The Magic and Making of Candles and Soaps

Days and Times of Power

Crossing The Third Threshold

How to Create a Magical Working Group

An Insider's Guide to the General Hospital Fan Club Weekend

Leaving Kentucky in the Broad Daylight

Real Magic

Get Your Book Published

Goddess in the Kitchen: The Magic and Making of Food

The Daughters of Avalon (Part of the Seven Sisters of Avalon Series)

Rose of Avalon (Part of the Seven Sisters of Avalon Series)

Where the Daffodils Grow(a novelette)